Aging Well is a treasure h :e
regarding how to live well, .re
they take a foothold on you, extend your precious years on earth, and
eventually die gracefully without much suffering. Dr. Venkit Iyer
discusses the role of 'nature' or genetic influences and 'nurture' or
habits and lifestyle, in achieving longevity. You have the power and
the passion to live your healthiest life possible and this book will help
you achieve just that. This s a must-read book for everybody.

**M. P. Ravindra Nathan, MD, FACC, FACP, FRCP
(London and Canada), FAHA Cardiologist, Emeritus Editor of AAPI
Journal, Author of *Stories from My Heart* and *Second Chance- A Sister's
Act of* Love**

This book encapsulates essential information to confront the
inevitable aging process. It lists practical steps to make it an enjoyable
and meaningful journey. Coming from a physician it addresses issues
of health, death, and also how to empower a surrogate to carry out
your wishes when you are no longer around or have become unable
to do so. A must-read book for everyone fortunate enough to reach
their golden years. Congratulations to Dr. Iyer for discussing essential
topics many individuals are too often reluctant to confront.

**Rajkumar K Warrier, MD, FACP. Gastroenterologist,
Author of *A Doctor's Odyssey: An Ode to Healing God***

Man's journey takes him through the ebb and flow of emotions,
intrigues, and the various vicissitudes of life. In the end, he needs to
know that he has arrived and the journey can be meticulously
planned by following Dr. Iyer's guidelines. A retired surgeon, Dr. Iyer
has first-hand knowledge of life, living, death, and dying. His book is
a comprehensive compilation of his personal observations and
experiences of life's journey and its inevitable conclusion.
Interspersed with anecdotes and stories he has put together an
impressive array of interesting topics. By living a healthier life, it is
possible to plan its end and die with dignity, knowing that one "has
arrived".

**Neria Harish Hebbar, MD, FACS.
General and Colorectal surgeon**

Aging Well and Reaching Beyond is a book about health and wellness and maintaining the best You possible. This book was written by a retired board-certified medical doctor of many years. All references to events, organizations, governments, persons, or locals are intended only to show multiple options and ideas on the topics of this book giving the reader the information to choose the paths and beliefs that work best for them. The information in this book is intended to be educational and used as an adjunct to a rational and responsible healthcare program and is not intended to replace professional medical advice. Any use of the information in this book is at the reader's discretion. The author and publisher disclaim any liability in connection with the use of this book.

Library of Congress Control Number: 2020949973

Published by Evershine Press, Inc.
1971 W Lumsden Rd #209
Brandon, FL 33511

ISBN: 978-0-9975108-6-7
eBook ISBN: 978-0-9975108-7-4

First edition: 2020

Printed in the United States of America

Table of Contents

About The Book

This book is about life. Birth and death are miracles. Codes are preset inside the genes of one single cell which can differentiate to all different organs, grow them to maturity and finally stop them from functioning. Death is inevitable. Between birth and death, a person's journey goes through multiple phases of joy and turmoil, uncertainty and surprises, ups and downs. While death is unavoidable, one can take efforts to postpone the eventuality, and enjoy the living period in the best way possible. How to live well, how to age gracefully, how to maintain good health, how to prepare oneself for the eventuality, and how to pass away peacefully? Most of the measures described are scientific ways that help one to undertake the journey well and end it nicely. This book describes wellness measures, preventive health care measures, care of the elderly, and planning for the end. It also goes over the science of death, dying with dignity, and the prevention of premature death. Finally, some thoughts are raised about immortality and life after death. The author sincerely hopes this book will be of value to many readers.

Foreword

by Kedambady P. Sheka, M.D., FACS

Dr. Venkit Iyer has done me a great honor a second time in a short period by requesting me to write a foreword to his second book. His first book, *Decision Making in Clinical Surgery* was written for medical professionals. I am happy to note the book was well received by young and old surgeons alike.

This present book, *Aging Well and Reaching Beyond* deals with a difficult subject. I am quite convinced Dr. Iyer is well prepared, for only he can put the reader at ease by his special style of presentation making the subject readable and enjoyable. This is a must-read book for all seniors and near retirement age adults. The breadth of reach of this writing surprises me; it seems like it has covered all the range of topics that are informative so you can have some peace of mind.

As science charges forward in all directions, it will face philosophical fronts from time to time. As man developed his inquisitive mind, he could not explain certain things by his reasoning on many occasions. He left that explanation to a Superior being. Dr. Iyer has handled several of these collusion points with extreme dexterity. He has quoted scriptures on many occasions, but at the same time, he has not taken the liberty to state them as facts. I guess the scientific enquiring mind in him lets him go only so far. I for one very much appreciate that.

I whole-heartedly endorse this masterful dissertation to the general public for its free-flowing style and content. From Dr.

Iyer's armamentarium, we should expect many more public interest volumes similar to this, to come out in the future. Wishing my long-time trusted friend and colleague every success.

Kedambady P. Sheka, MD, FACS
Retd. Chairman of Surgical services, Coney Island Hospital,
Brooklyn, New York-11235

Dedication

I dedicate this book to my Parents, Mentors, Teachers, Family, and Friends.

Acknowledgment

I wish to thank Evershine Press, Inc and Ms. Jewel Parago for their excellent work in getting this book published. Without their valuable help in editing, proofreading, formatting, and printing this book I would not have been able to complete this project. My sincere thanks to Ms. Jewel Parago, who is a wonderful person.

I wish to thank Dr. Kedambady Sheka, who is retired Chairman of the Department of Surgery at Coney Island Hospital in New York for reviewing the book, making valuable suggestions, and writing a forward message. I also wish to thank Dr. M.P. Ravindra Nathan, Dr. Rajkumar Warrier, and Dr. Neria Harish Hebbar for taking the time to review the draft copy of the book, making suggestions and for writing positive remarks and providing encouragement. All of them are physicians of high standards and achievements and I value their support.

I must also thank my family and many friends who have given me encouragement, suggestions, and support in my endeavor. I hope the readers will benefit from some of my narratives.

Preface

This is a book about aging and dying. How to age well and how to die well? While both are inevitable, one can prepare for the best scenario.

The number of people reaching 100 years old is expected to reach an all-time high by the next 10 years. People are living longer and this has its good and bad sides. This book hopes to address some of the issues of aging well while maintaining good health.

How to have a good life, how to live well, how to be happy, how to avoid premature death, and eventually how to die gracefully? Immortality may be a dream, but we have prolonged life and postponed death. We continue to do so. Each day we live we have postponed death by that day, but we are also getting closer to death by one day. Wellness measures, good living, preventive medical care, treatment of medical problems in a timely and appropriate fashion, and avoiding unnecessary risks are ways to increase longevity.

Death is a morbid and unwelcome topic for most people. It is depressing and uncomfortable to discuss this subject for many people. However, death is inevitable. Everyone will certainly die. However, there is an innate desire for all biological creatures to avoid death and live as long as possible. Humans are no exception.

From time immemorial, the search for immortality has been described and the search continues even today. While it has not been possible to avoid death altogether, success has been accomplished in postponing the eventual day, by nearly doubling the life expectancy of humans over the past 200 years.

Hindu mythology describes a potion or nectar called "Amritam". If it is taken by mouth, the person becomes immortal and goes to heaven. Christians believe that Jesus Christ was resurrected from death. The mythology goes that those who drink from the chalice that was used for the last supper by Jesus Christ will attain immortality. The search for that chalice continues even today. The Greeks believed in an unseen, mysterious fountain of youth, which gave life-sustaining water ensuring youth forever.

From ancient civilizations to modern-day religions, many believe that there is life after death. The soul departs from the worn-out body, but the soul is immortal. We discard worn-out cloth and wear a new one. If the person was good-natured during earthly life, the soul goes to heaven. If the person was evil-minded then the soul goes to hell for perpetual punishment. Either way, there is a continuation of life beyond the planet earth. Whether there is truth in this assumption or not is open for argument. However, it does help to inculcate moral values and decent life encouraging many thousands to lead a good life out of fear or reward.

What causes death, how is death defined, when is death confirmed, what should we do upon the death of our dear one, and funeral arrangements are different items that deserve discussion.

How to prepare for the end of life, what are the legal details to be addressed before death, Living Will, durable power of attorney, will for one's estate, estate planning, and life insurance are another set of issues.

Dying with dignity and comfort, avoiding the miserable last few days, and having family nearby are some things most of us want. What is Hospice care, what are comfort measures, and how do they differ from physician-assisted suicide? What is the role of organ transplantation and how do your tissues live for a longer time in another person's body?

Also, we need to address the prevention of death in young people in the prime their of lives. This includes reducing gun violence, reducing drug addiction, reducing accidents, suicides, and homicides.

Immortality is a dream, a myth, and impractical. If all those who are born continue to live forever, the planet would be overcrowded. Birth and death are part of a cycle.

In modern-day, immortality means living well for as long as possible, and not living forever. Despite all the progress we have made, it is still difficult to define the exact moment and time life begins and the exact moment and time when life ends. We make approximations. However, everyone born must die one day and there is no escape for anyone.

This is a book about life and death. To understand death, we need to understand birth. Where does life begin and where does it end? What is the path God has destined for us? Can we alter Nature? There is much emotion, consternation, agony, and happiness that flows through the life of a person. Biological science and genetic science have made remarkable progress in the past decade. We know that life is DNA, and DNA is a set of chemicals carrying certain codes. Still, we cannot make new life de-novo in the laboratory out of those chemicals, and yet we do not know why it stops functioning one day.

I sincerely hope this book will provide some guidance and provoke some thoughts to my readers.

Section-1 Living Well

Chapter-1

THE PROCESS OF AGING

When I ask the age of my grandson who is 4 years old, he will usually say "I am four and a half years old". When you are young, you cannot wait to get older. You wish you were older and independent so you can do many things that adults do. You are in a hurry to get older, so you can drive a car, go the movies, watch PG 13 movies, build up muscles, or go out on a date, and so forth.

Once you get older, you wish you were younger. When asked your age, you like to state it one year younger than you are. You want to dye your hair, have some plastic surgery to remove the wrinkles, drive a fancy car, or dress like a chic. One day it hits you suddenly that you are getting older. Till then you think you are still young and you have all the time the world to achieve and conquer. For some, it is the 40th birthday as they call it the big 40. For some others, it may be 65 when Medicare calls you over the phone to set up a phone interview. For still some others, it is when others call you "Uncle" or "Sir" or even as "Grand Pa".

Aging can be chronological stating the actual number of years you have lived or it can be biological reflecting the state of health that equates you to one comparable. A young person can be physiologically older due to medical problems, obesity, or addictive habits and poor lifestyle. Also, older people can feel and look younger if they do not have these issues. All of us want to live well, feel well, with a good quality of life up to the very end.

Whether we like it or not, aging happens. We are all on a one-way conveyor belt, like the luggage coming out of an airplane. They go only forwards, and not backward. Some of the luggage may fall off the belt; some will reach the end of the line. Aging is one way only, it can only go forward with time, and never backward. Some people will fall off and die on the way, some others will live longer and yet a few others will live to their fullest.

Another way to describe it is "rivers do not reverse". A river flows towards the ocean. The water flows only down and further down, it can never flow reverse. Life is like a leaf floating in the water. Some leaves float to a certain distance and wash ashore. Some go for further down and some eventually reach the ocean. You cannot get back the time or the age that has become the past.

The main reason for aging is genetic and we may not have much control over it. Just look at the skin and subcutaneous tissue of a five and a fifty-year-old. The face of the five-year-old is chubby, full, and shiny. Pinch it, and it fills back instantly. It is hard to find a vein in the arm or leg. The fifty-year-old has loose skin, with wrinkles settling in, and bags are beginning to form under the chin or the eyes. Pinching the skin here, you will see it is so loose and it takes longer to return to normalcy. It is easy to find veins in the wrist, forearms, and legs. What happened in the intervening period? The skin lost its collagen and elastin in the connective tissue, in the process of aging. This is just one of the manifestations of aging.

Human cells wear out and die after a while. Cumulative wear and tear occur. It may be those energy molecules called ATP that become lower. It may be that oxygen molecules allow "free radicals" to form, which prevents the electronic equilibrium to be maintained. Telomeres that represent the DNA pattern in the chromosomes get shortened and break off, which in turn leads to the death of the cell.

Aging Well and Reaching Beyond

Aging may be due to two aspects: Nature or nurture. Nature is a genetic influence and nurture is the environmental influence. Scientists believe that we are genetically programmed to age and die. Individual cells in the body have different life spans. Hundreds of thousands of our cells die daily, but we reproduce them also. Stomach cells last about 2 days, red blood cells last 120 days, bone cells last for 30 years, and so forth. Despite the reformation of cells, the body as a whole is slated to slow down and become weak. Different living species have different life spans built into their genetic code. Houseflies live for 35 days, while a sequoia tree lives for 2500 years. Humans live for 100 years.

The second cause of aging has to do with Nurture: of our own making, due to our lifestyle and outlook. Some of these items are further detailed in the section of "Wellness". These are items one can control, unlike the natural aging process. With attention to these details along with progress in science and medicine, we have already doubled the life expectancy of the human population over the past 200 years. Humans may likely live to 120 years routinely in the next 200 years. 80 and 90 years old's may not be old then.

As the time comes for retirement, many are at a loss. Having worked long hours and being actively engaged, suddenly the emptiness and lack of activity can be troublesome. The Japanese say that a couple has more friction, divorce, and suicide after retirement. However, there is life after retirement and it can be enjoyable as well. One just needs to plan activities to fill the day and keep engaged in worldly affairs.

Look at the benefits of becoming a senior citizen. One gets Medicare health insurance that covers 80% of their medical expenses. For the remaining 20%, one can sign up with a supplemental insurance policy or simply join a Medicare Advantage plan, which takes over 100% of medical expenses. Social security starts coming in, and for many people, it is a big relief. Even though it may not cover all expenses, it does help to bridge the gap for many families. Then there are many senior citizen discounts and perks, from movie tickets to airline travel. My barbershop gives a 10% discount for seniors for a haircut. Admission to theme parks and food in certain restaurants are also discounted for seniors.

Seniors get more respect and admiration in Eastern cultures. This may not be so evident in Western society. In Japan, China, and India seniors and elders are honored and respected in their homes as well as in places of gathering or festivities. They are given preferred seating and given proper recognition. They are looked upon as a source of wisdom, advice, and fairness. Family members ask their opinion and blessings before finalizing weddings, jobs, and real estate investments.

This is somewhat different in the Western Hemisphere. Older people are often seen as a burden to the family and society. Very elderly are at times ignored as useless, requiring care and attention. They are not given jobs even if they are capable of doing so. The status of the elderly reached a low point during the Great Depression. The value of a member is measured by their ability to be productive in earning income. They were often neglected and even abused. Many elderly die alone in a nursing home or adult care centers even though they have families. They do not want to provide care for the old and incapacitated ones at their homes as they do in the Eastern culture.

To maintain a certain level of self-respect it is important for the elderly to remain affluent and wealthy, to be healthy and independent as long as possible. As one gets older, they generally become wiser, softer, and more tolerant compared to their own younger age. They also tend to believe in God, destiny and cherish family and friends.

Staying in good health is certainly more of a priority, more than being wealthy for the elderly.

There are numerous forms of advice from advertisements, books, TV programs, and others to tell you what you should and should not be doing to remain healthy. With good health comes independence, and self-esteem. There are many offers and discounts for joining health clubs, to follow diet regimens, and about senior active daycare programs. Dietary regimens are filled with measurement of calories, vitamins, anti-oxidants, probiotics, turmeric, and whole milk. Weight loss programs, pretty bodies, muscular chests, vigor in sex, memory power, and success in life are offered for you by simply subscribing to a certain liquid formula.

Essentially, we are looking forward to "Healthy Aging" instead of just aging. Healthy aging involves (1) Low numbers of illnesses and disabilities (2) High cognitive and physical functioning, and (3) Active engagement with life. Examples are activities such as traveling, independent living, driving, participation in sports or group activities, managing financial affairs, and enjoying fine arts.

Life expectancy in Japan is 84 as the world's highest. 28% of the Japanese people are over 65, in comparison with 15% in the USA. This also means higher expenses for health care and elder care by the government. The government tries its best to control health care costs by setting fee schedules, and denying unnecessary tests and procedures, and encouraging home health care. Other measures include raising the retirement age and providing preventive care and community services.

In summary, aging is a natural process and it is unstoppable since time only moves forward. The question is how long one can remain in good health and be independent and not a question of how many years one remains alive.

Chapter-2

WELLNESS MEASURES

Postponing death or prevention of premature death is the same as increasing longevity. It translates as a step towards immortality. Many of the items described in this chapter are common sense issues, but they will help one to maintain good mental and physical health. Good health leads to prolonging life and postponing death. These are called as wellness measures and consist of simple attention to lifestyle issues.

From prehistoric times, generations of people all over the world have wanted to live longer and healthier. Therefore, it is no wonder that patients ask for advice to prevent a heart attack, stroke, and to have a healthy life. Much of the discussion is good for the prevention of atherosclerosis, falls, depression, and dementia, and cancer.

Diet: An ancient Greek physician Hippocrates said in the 4th century BC, "Let food be your medicine". Food can be considered as a medicine for many illnesses. This still holds.

The amount of food consumed, the number of calories, types of food and drinks, provide the necessary components such as vitamins, minerals, and proteins, and avoidance of harmful food items are all various factors to be considered. Commercial firms have developed technology to identify DNA markers that will give personalized advice on the best foods to consume for good health.

Types of food: The Mediterranean diet is considered to be one of the best examples of a good diet. It consists of vegetables, lentils, beans, nuts, fruits, fish, or fish oil supplements, and olive oil. It is best to avoid fatty and greasy foods, sugary items, animal fats, and red meat.

Unhealthy diets are red meat items such as barbequed beef, hamburgers and cheeseburgers, french fries, donuts, pastries and cakes, potato chips, and cola drinks. Type 2 diabetes can be controlled with diet by reducing carbohydrates such as rice, bread, and sweets and by medications.

A randomized clinical trial of 48,000 women conducted by the Women's Health initiative in 2019 confirmed that postmenopausal women have a reduced risk of dying from breast cancer if they followed a low-fat diet with fruits, vegetables, and grains compared to those who had a high-fat diet with non-vegetarian foods.

Similarly, dietary control is effective against hypertension, heart diseases, stroke, diabetes mellitus, other types of cancers such as pancreatic, gastric, colorectal, and hepatic, and such visceral malignancies on prior studies.

Research published in the Journal of the American Medical Association in 2019 found that consumption of two or more glasses of soft drinks with sugar or artificial sweeteners was associated with death from various causes including circulatory problems and digestive diseases. The study was based on 451,743 men and women from 10 European countries, surveying their food and drink consumption. Participants who had prior illnesses such as heart diseases, stroke, diabetes mellitus, and cancers were excluded from the study. Heavy soft drink consumption leads to higher BMI (Body mass index) and also tend to be smokers.

Reduce salt: Avoiding extra salt is a good measure in reducing heart attacks, reducing clogged arteries, and improving kidney function. Dr. Surender Reddy Neravetla has written a book, "Salt Kills" and he gives numerous talks on the adverse effects of excess salt in daily food. He recommends the removal of salt and pepper shakers from dining tables altogether.

Quality: Omega 3 fatty acids are good to reduce blood pressure and plaque buildup inside arteries. Omega 3 fatty acids are found in fish or fish oil. Those who are total vegetarians can get this supplement in a pill form. Antioxidants can fight to slow the growth of cancer and increase the longevity of cells. They have anti-aging properties when one considers oxidation as a cause of cell death. They are found in blueberries, strawberries, and fresh fruits. Glucosinolates convert to compounds that slow the growth of cancer cells. They are found in broccoli and other green vegetables. Nuts and seeds can repair chromosomes, allowing the cells to live longer. Polyphenols found in apples can slow the growth of cancer cells. Berries increase memory power and delay the onset of dementia. Cranberry juice, pomegranate juice, and red wine have resveratrol in them that reduces heart attacks and cholesterol build up inside arteries.

Antioxidants: Oxidation occurs when the cells become destabilized and leads to the formation of free radicals. Excess accumulation of free radicals causes cell deterioration and eventual cell death. Antioxidants reduce the free radical formation and thus prolong cell life. Antioxidants are good for reducing illnesses and improving healthier life. Antioxidants are found in plenty of food items that cover the colors of the rainbow. They are seen in fresh fruits of all types, berries such as blueberry, strawberry, raspberry, vegetables such as carrots, sweet potato, beets, beans, green vegetables such as broccoli, cabbage, spinach, pecan nuts, red tomatoes, red cabbage, eggplants, and turmeric. In other words, most fresh vegetables, fresh fruits, and nuts are good for the body.

Fiber: It is good to have fiber in the diet because it provides volume in the stomach filling one up, and has less sugary counterparts as compared to refined carbohydrates. Fiber allows food to be digested slowly with fewer fluctuations in sugar level in the blood. Fiber also allows one to eat with fewer calories compared to items such as donuts and pastries. It reduces constipation and straining by adding bulk to stool.

Supplements: One has to focus on getting all the various minerals, vitamins, proteins, and essential fatty acids along with carbohydrates when planning a diet. Ancient Indian food items that include turmeric, ginger, and spices combined to make sauces like "Sambar" is healthy. So are ancient diets from Japan and China. Citrus fruits have vitamin C, spinach has iron, and fresh fruits have other vitamins.

Quantity: Quantity should be controlled to avoid obesity. One method is to stop eating once the stomach is three-quarters full by avoiding that last serving. Slowly the stomach size shrinks and the quantity of food slowly comes down over a while. Another method is called 'partial fasting'. Here one is fasting for an extra few hours before the food is taken. Initially, the stomach will growl and one can drink some water. Slowly the time interval between food intakes is increased from four hours to six hours and then to eight hours and the craving for food and hunger pains subsides. During the Ramadan month, Muslims do not eat for twelve hours during the daytime for a whole month. Hindus observe night fasting on several occasions throughout the year, particularly on new moon days, death anniversary days of ancestors, and other religious holidays.

Another way to reduce the quantity of food is to eat slowly and in smaller amounts of food in each mouth full. Chew the food as long as possible, savor the taste, and take your time before swallowing it before putting the next scoop of food into your mouth. Slow eating reduces the total intake. Do not hurry up and swallow big chunks and large quantities

Calories: Calorie count is checked to avoid excessive calories per day. One way to reduce calories is to take green leaves and vegetables that are filling as opposed to sugary food and excess carbohydrates. Fruits and nuts are better used as snacks instead of bread, candies, muffins, and donuts. Water or fruit juices are used instead of cola drinks or sugary drinks.

Avoid sugary desserts such as ice cream, puddings, cakes and instead have fresh fruits or skip the dessert altogether.

Exercise: Regular exercise of any type is very helpful to maintain joint flexibility and muscle strength. It reduces obesity and reduces atherosclerosis plaque buildup. It can be any form of exercise such as simple walking, swimming, running or a workout in the gymnasium or it can consist of participation in a sporting activity such as tennis, golf, basketball, soccer, or hockey. Stretching exercises as in yoga, karate, Tai chi or pull-ups and push-ups are fine too. One must have a routine built into daily or weekly schedules. Dancing, skiing, figure skating can be fun combined with music. Regular exercises keeps the body fit and trim, reduces weight, reduces the chance of obesity, improves social interactions especially in team sports, keeping the blood pressure low, and reduces the chance of atherosclerosis. Endorphin, which is a happiness hormone flows during exercises and keeps the person in a comfortable state called 'the zone'. This allows peace and stress reduction, thus prolonging life and ensuring a healthier life. Exercise not only improves physical fitness; it also improves brainpower.

Exercise does not always mean sweaty, puffing, and straining strenuous activity. New federal guidelines state that many less obvious movements can also be considered exercise such as activities that include climbing the stairs instead of taking the elevator, raking the leaves, mowing the lawn, cleaning the patio, walking short distances at the workplace, shopping at the grocery store, cleaning the house, dancing, gardening, bicycling for short distances instead of driving the car and so forth. Every movement counts, such as standing, walking while making phone calls, and standing in the subway or bus. These light activities are called NEAT (non-exercise activity thermogenesis) and can become supplementary to more vigorous activities for at least an hour or two per week. The new slogan is "move more, sit less".

Obesity prevention: Obesity is proven to be a health hazard, which leads to a variety of medical problems and hastens death. It causes early onset of diabetes mellitus, osteoporosis, lung problems, heart problems, skin ulcerations, and eventually reduces life expectancy by 30 years. Obese people have a great deal of difficulty in losing weight despite all efforts. About 40% of Americans are obese, and as obesity becomes more common there is less motivation for people to lose weight. The best option is to stay slim from childhood and keep the lower weight throughout one's life, with proper diet and exercise. Obese individuals must consult a physician for therapy. There are specialist physicians for obesity management; weight watchers as they are called. The initial emphasis is on dietary control. Various dietary regimens are described. It is important to lose weight slowly, with attention to vitamins, trace elements, essential amino acids, and essential fatty acids. If dietary control fails, the next best option is to have surgery. Many different surgical procedures have been tried. The latest preference appears to be laparoscopic sleeve gastrectomy, with or without robotic assistance.

Stress reduction: Stress, anxiety, and isolation can herald the onset of mental depression and inaction. Having a family, social activities, friends, group activities of any kind, visiting places of worship, meditation, and yoga are useful methods. One will have to analyze our reasons for stress and write them down. This will help to overcome the stress points. If it is caused by multitasking, stop the same activities, and take one thing at a time. Maybe it's due to a lack of sleep. Arrange an adequate time for rest and relaxation. A certain amount of time is needed to take care of children and their requirements. Stress may be due to pressure at work, either excessive work, inability to meet the competition or discrimination. It may be due to marital issues, divorce, or separation.

Scientific evidence shows that stress is harmful to health. Heart rate goes up, blood pressure goes up, and breathing becomes rapid and labored. The whole body internally and externally gets tensed up with increased adrenaline flow. Behavioral changes occur with anger and irritation leading to verbal or physical reactions. There is an increased chance of heart attack and stroke. The digestive system shuts down with episodes of nausea or vomiting. Mental faculty is affected causing errors, memory loss, an inability to focus, and job performance suffers. Headaches, asthma, hysteria, and temper tantrums can lead to work delinquencies. Social and physical wellness is affected by stress.

Nowadays we are spending too much time on cell phones, computers, and televisions resulting in less direct interaction with people. It is estimated that we are looking at a digital screen during 50% of our awake hours for one reason or another. There is pressure to check the cell phone for messages constantly. Social media is a big culprit here. Stop looking at the cellphone constantly and stop the urge to read and reply to messages instantly. They can wait- often it is something silly. The person on the cell phone seems to get more attention than the person sitting in front of you at the dinner table. When talking to someone, look into their eyes instead of looking at the cell phone.

It is good to learn some relaxation techniques to reduce stress. Take a few minutes off from the table when tired. Walk or talk. Have a cup of coffee or tea. Take a deep breath and do some deep breathing exercises or stretching exercises. Take a power nap. It will do wonders. Meditation and Yoga are other methods that help.

Uncorrected stress can lead to depression. At this point, one should seek medical advice. One may need counseling or medications. If left uncorrected it can lead to further mental disorders or suicides.

Mental tasks: Keeping the brain engaged will reduce the onset of dementia and will help the growth of new neuronal cells. Mental work can be in different forms, such as playing board games, reading, writing, teaching, arts and crafts, chess, crossword puzzle, Sudoku, and working. Simply reading daily newspaper keeps one in touch with the local and national events, improves vocabulary, and keeps the brain engaged. Join a book club and discuss a book that you recently read. New neurons sprout by keeping the brain active by thinking, learning, and challenging it regularly. This is proven by MRI scans, showing increased gray matter and increased activity in the brain on those who challenge their minds at least two hours each day.

Mental depression, dementia, and neurological disorders such as Alzheimer's disease may be related to aging, but they may also be related to illnesses, addictions, or correctable socio-economic issues.

Sex: Touch is one of the five senses, the other senses being taste, smell, vision, and hearing. Eating delicious food, listening to good music, seeing nature and beauty, and smelling good odors bring peace and happiness. Touching, cuddling, and good sex also provide happiness, contentment, meaning in life, and improve social interaction and friendship. The Oxytocin hormone is a happy hormone and is associated with the normal biology of pregnancy and childbearing. The baby wants to be held, it stops crying and smiles when it is held. So do the adults. Kissing, holding hands, touching each other may or may not lead to sex, but it is certainly one of the wellness measures that improves good health, both mentally and physically. One can see a certain glow and contentment in the eyes of happily married people. Married people live longer and healthier than singles.

Sleep: Sleep requirements can vary, but on average, one should get seven hours of sleep per night. It is enviable to be able to sleep well because it provides good rest to the body and mind. It is very refreshing the next day for activities. The brain needs time off, and sleep is part of the brain's biorhythm. Older people are unable to sleep soundly as the younger ones do. Inadequate sleep leads to a variety of medical problems and accelerates the aging process. Insomnia is a medical problem for several people. Watching less television, light meals, reading a book, and at times sleeping pills are methods that induce sleep. During sleep hours, the body and brain regenerate the tissues, heals the cells, and replaces the lost cells. Growth hormones are secreted during sleep, allowing youngsters to grow while they sleep. The immune system gets recharged, melatonin is secreted and neurons get needed rest for regeneration. Sleep deprivation causes various physical and mental problems, starting from irritability to instability and irrationality to unconsciousness. Unexplained weight gain is another side effect. About 20% of all road accidents are related to tiredness and sleeping while driving. Other side effects of inadequate sleep are confusion, memory loss, poor concentration, mood changes, clumsiness, frequent sicknesses, high blood pressure, type 2 diabetes mellitus, weight gain, low sex drive, infertility, heart disease, injuries, low athletic performance, short temper, a higher chance of stroke, dangerous driving, under-eye bags, dehydration, under-eye circles, and lower skills leading to errors at the workplace.

Addictive habits: Avoid certain addictive habits such as smoking, chewing tobacco, snuff, and excess use of alcohol. Avoid addictive drugs such as painkillers, Percocet, and Oxycontin. Avoid street drugs such as cocaine, heroin, and synthetic drugs. A small amount of alcohol in moderation is acceptable. Some studies show that red wine may reduce the chance of heart attacks or atherosclerotic plaque buildup through resveratrol, a chemical in wine, and other foods. Cranberry juice and pomegranate juice are also thought to be beneficial. Do not mix alcohol with sleeping pills, sedatives, opioid drugs. Do not get into binge drinking.

Dental hygiene: Routine dental care gets less attention in third world countries. Good dental hygiene prevents many oral cavity problems as well as systemic problems. Flossing should be done regularly after every meal and brushing should be done twice daily. It also improves social interactions and mental confidence. Good dental condition is an indicator of good habits, good hygiene, and good health.

Safety: Prevention of accidents, injuries, and falls is critical. Most of the trauma admissions to hospitals today are related to falls and accidents. Many surgical procedures and resulting side effects can be avoided simply by being careful. They also include avoiding pollutants of various natures from the air, water, food, and noise. Safe sex and the use of condoms can prevent sexually transmitted diseases. The use of seat belts and airbags have reduced automobile accidents considerably. Helmets must be worn while driving bicycles or two-wheelers such as scooters, motorcycles, or while skiing, rollerblading, or snowboarding. Avoid the use of cell phones in any fashion while driving. Texting while driving is dangerous and illegal in many states.

Medical checkups and disease management: Control of known chronic medical conditions such as diabetes mellitus, hypertension, respiratory problems, allergic conditions, neurological, or urological problems is preventative health care. It is good to have a family doctor who can do routine physical examinations and various tests to ensure good health. Early detection of abnormalities with corrective steps can prevent many complications, and lives can be saved and premature deaths avoided. Routine blood tests will detect anemia, chronic blood loss, nutritional deficiencies, blood cancers, diabetes, kidney disease, cholesterol levels, and lipids profile, cancers, liver disorders, and certain metabolic disorders. These could go undetected otherwise until an advanced situation arises which could be life-threatening. Very often these could be corrected by taking medications or supplements.

Looking good is feeling good: Good grooming, cleanliness, facial hygiene, eyebrows, attire, skin and hair conditioning, and a good smile are all good things, which bring in good company, better social activity, and personal self-confidence and self-esteem. All of these lead to feeling good, which translates to a better mental state and better health. Moisturizing skin cream helps to avoid dryness of the skin. Dry skin can lead to itching and scratching, which in turn causes small ulcerations and skin infections. It also causes more skin wrinkling. Properly fitting shoes for walking as well as for different sporting activities is important to reduce falls and ankle and foot injuries. Showering or bathing twice a day reduces surface infections, and proper hair grooming reduces scalp infestations with lice and ticks. Body odor can be repulsive and it is good to use deodorants.

Independence: Loss of independence is one of the scariest events for an older person. As one loses hearing, vision, cognition, and balance, it becomes necessary to depend on others for daily functions. It becomes quite disheartening, especially when one's mind is still agile. Eight items on the checklist to determine physical independence are the ability to use the toilet, eating, dressing, bathing, grooming, getting out of bed, getting out of a chair, and walking. Eight items on the checklist for independent living are the ability to do shopping, cooking, housekeeping, handle financial matters, do laundry, make phone calls, travel, and take medications. Driving is an added boost. Independence gives mental comfort and strength.

Hobbies: It is good to nurture a hobby because it brings satisfaction, fun, and relaxation. It makes one age slower than they otherwise would. It allows one to interact with others, and pleasantly exercise the body and brain. It encourages one to focus and learn new skills, thus allowing the brain to make new neurons. Hobbies are something you like to do for fun besides your work, thus reducing work-related stress. This can be any activity you like to do, possibly a form of exercise or sporting activity or something creative like carpentry or architecture or building. Maybe art such as painting, music, reading, writing, photography, pottery, sculpting, dancing, or acting. Even volunteering to help others or going to church or hospital. Games such as bridge, card games, chess, or board games. Whatever it may be, it should be something you enjoy and something you share with others. If you can share it with your spouse or family members it adds to your bonding.

Happiness and Peace: According to the Dalai Lama, happiness is a state of the mind. In other words, it has to come from within you. Some people are never going to be happy no matter how much they own and how much they get. They keep comparing themselves to others. Those who are happy live longer; have less stress and fewer diseases.

About half of the happiness a person has is an inborn habit, about 10% is due to circumstances, and the remaining 40% is based on one's attitude. This last group can make an effort and make themselves happier by taking the right steps in their outlook. Instead of looking at negatives all the time, they could look at some of the positives. Smiling more often and by making small talks with strangers and customers will increase friends. Avoiding controversial topics such as politics or personal matters will reduce tension. Counting one's blessings in life, and recognizing one's errors committed in the past will bring in peace. Finally accepting destiny or fate or God's will instead of taking the blame on themselves for events that get out of control will reduce mental stress.

Money helps a person up to a certain level, to feel secure and comfortable, but beyond a certain level, it does not increase happiness. Too much money brings more stress and addictive habits and eventual unhappiness. Social activities, volunteerism, enjoying nature, personal accomplishments, and activities are ways to improve happiness level.

There are four happiness hormones described that can bring in contentment. Endorphin is an activity hormone. Exercise in any form allows this to be secreted into the blood, making one feel better. Laughter also raises endorphin levels. Dopamine is an achievement hormone that makes one feel good when a difficult task is achieved or a test is passed. When someone recognizes your efforts or praises your achievements, the dopamine level can go up. Serotonin is a socializing hormone that makes one feel better when having friends, social conversations, and group activities. Finally, oxytocin is a touch hormone that makes one feel good even with a simple touch. A crying baby stops crying when held.

Five sensations that we know namely taste, smell, hearing, seeing, and touch also brings in good feelings. Tasting good food or drink, smelling good perfume or flowers, listening to good music, reading a good book or watching a sunset and birds, and hugging and holding the hands of a good friend or spouse, holding grandchildren in your lap are all items that bring in happiness, smiling and good feelings. Most of these things are inexpensive, they are free for you to enjoy.

Prayer, Meditation: Placing the belief in supreme power, praying to one's chosen God or following religious rituals, and meditating in any fashion are tools available for one to find peace and calm. It may not be for everyone and many may not believe in these rituals. However, if it works for someone, that person should continue to seek such solace. Irrespective of God or religion, three tenets to follow as per ancient scriptures to live in peace are 1. Cause no harm to others: such harm could be caused by one's deeds, words, or even thoughts. 2. Help someone if you can, and care about others. 3. Accept that the world is chaotic and learn to live in this world the way it is.

Meditation is a form of relaxation of the mind and body. It requires some amount of willful effort to control an overactive mind while the thoughts jump through various bits and pieces. It can be practiced at any time anywhere. It calms the mind from anxiety, impatience, reduces stress, and anger. It helps to lower blood pressure, anxiety, chronic pain syndromes, and thus increases longevity and youthfulness.

Nature: Mother Nature is kind and good to all. It is free for enjoyment. Sunlight is good for the skin and helps to generate vitamin D. One should be careful in avoiding too much sunlight and the use of sunscreen and hats are recommended. Waterfronts make us feel peaceful and calm. We are water born animals by evolution, we were in a medium of water in the mother's womb, and our body mass is 80% made of water. No wonder we feel attracted to a beachfront and waterfront whenever possible. Trees, gardens, flowers, lakes, rivers, mountains, green grass, butterflies, deer, snow, and glaciers are just some of the things that come with nature that make us smile and become happy. Being with nature is like being with God and being with Mother. In our daily hurry to make ends meet we often forget to enjoy what is there and free.

Nature provides good health and longevity. Avoiding pollution will improve health. In other words, those who live in polluted areas of the world lose their longevity. It was recently mentioned that those living in highly polluted areas such as New Delhi or Beijing are inhaling bad pollutants equivalent to smoking 50 cigarettes a day. They develop allergic reactions, asthma, and upper respiratory conditions.

There is no age limit to start any of these wellness measures. Often people say that they are too old to start these changes. Not true. One will see improvements as soon as one institutes these changes.

Chapter-3

CANCER SCREENING

Early detection of cancer has the best chance of cure. This is well proven in breast cancers, colorectal cancers, and skin cancers. Some of the cancers can probably be prevented from occurring by taking precautionary measures. For example, colonoscopy and removal of polyps can reduce the incidence of colorectal cancers; the use of sunscreens and avoiding exposure to the sun can reduce melanoma of the skin. Lifestyle habits such as diet, exercise, and avoidance of alcohol or smoking can reduce various malignancies. Screening for cancer and having regular medical checkups are good health measures.

"I want to know if I have cancer." Patients want this information often. Physicians are also supposed to do cancer screenings to diagnose and treat cancers early for a better outcome.

There is no single test for finding cancers. However, there are several steps one can take in preventative health care.

Skin- Early diagnosis of melanoma and squamous cell cancers can lead to curative treatments by simple wide local excisions. Once they are advanced, cure rates go down even after complex therapies. Patients and physicians are advised to have any and every abnormal-looking skin lesion examined, biopsied, or excised if necessary.

Protecting against sun exposure is a useful measure. One may avoid direct exposure to the sun, by applying sunscreen lotion, or covering up the body with clothing when outside.

Breast- Early diagnosis of breast cancer gives an almost 90% chance for a permanent cure. Routine physical examination, self-examination, and screening mammograms are the available tools. Those who have a family history of breast cancers or who had prior gynecological cancers are at a higher risk. Gene testing for BRCA gene mutations can be done for those at high risk.

Cervix- Routine pap smears and regular GYN checkups are useful tools. Abnormal menstrual cycles or flows are investigated. HPV (Human Papilloma Virus) vaccine can reduce the incidence of cervical cancer and head and neck cancers.

Lung- Avoid smoking habits at all costs. Also avoid pollution if possible, whether it is work-related or environment-related. Those who had exposure to asbestos and mining are at higher risk. Those at high risk can obtain a CT scan of the chest once every ten years. Obtain physical examination and tests upon noticing coughing spells or hemoptysis.

Colorectal- Report any change in bowel habits or rectal bleeding for further evaluation. Routine screening of the stool for microscopic blood by hemoccult testing is a good first step. Other tests of value are the FIT test (Fecal Immunoassay Test) for colonic blood and the Cologuard test, which uses DNA analysis of the stool for early cancers and polyps. A blood test for screening is also in the developmental stage. A screening colonoscopy once every ten years is recommended. Polyps diagnosed early can be removed by the endoscope, thus preventing cancer formation.

Prostate- A routine PSA (prostate-specific antigen) has certain advantages. A routine rectal examination and prostate ultrasound can be done to pick up occult lesions.

Lumps and bumps- All abnormal lumps and bumps should be evaluated. They could be enlarged lymph nodes, which could in turn be a spread from another source of cancer or a primary lymphoma.

Testicular- Routine physical examinations should include palpation of testes for tumors, hydrocele, and hernia. Patients are also to report any abnormalities.

Visceral malignancies- One must follow up on unexplained weight loss, loss of appetite, vomiting, abdominal pain, or vomiting blood. A complete physical examination and necessary tests that may include a CT scan or GI endoscopy are recommended.

Brain tumors- Do not ignore unusual headaches, visual or hearing disturbances, falls, blackouts, fainting spells, or balance problems. Consult a neurologist and obtain a CT scan or MRI of the brain.

Blood test- A regular complete blood count with peripheral smear can reveal leukemia, anemia, and bone marrow abnormalities. Certain markers for cancers such as CRP, Alpha-fetoproteins, Ca-19, and Ca-125 have been described but are not specific for a diagnosis. Newer efforts to find a genetic abnormality for cancer are being worked on.

Other steps- Exercise regularly, eat a healthy diet, avoid addictions to alcohol, avoid smoking and drugs, and live in a healthy neighborhood.

A routine physical examination by a primary care physician and routine tests to evaluate any unusual symptoms are recommended.

Venkit S. Iyer

Family history of cancers, history of previous cancers, history of exposure to cancerogenic agents, living in neighborhoods with pollutants, working in radiology, or nuclear-related fields are conditions that should raise the level of caution.

Chapter-4

MEDICAL BENEFITS OF YOGA

Yoga is getting more recognition as a meaningful preventative health care measure all over the world. United Nations recognized June 21st as International Yoga Day, and India observed the day with great fanfare.

There is a fair amount of confusion, vagueness, and misunderstanding about Yoga, especially on items relating to Ayurveda, and associated historic, religious, and socio-economic aspects.

When we mention the word yoga many things flash through our mind. Is it the mystic man in a faraway forest hiding in hibernation or is it the yoga studio in your community where skinny girls in tight yoga pants take up pretzel-like postures? Is it a holistic or nature therapy or is it a commercialized hoax?

What is the real scientific value of yoga? What are the facts versus fiction? What are the medically proven true benefits of yoga?

When we inspect closely on the nuts and bolts of it, we recognize three main medical components of Yoga, namely breathing exercises, stretching exercises, and meditation practices.

Breathing Exercises: Breathing is part of life. We breathe regularly, without even knowing that we are breathing. So how can it become an exercise?

We can voluntarily regulate breathing as a useful tool for achieving a relaxed state and clear mind along with certain physical benefits.

Several things happen when one takes a deep breath slowly, holds it for a few seconds, and exhales it slowly. Automatically our posture becomes more erect, and the chest, abdominal, and diaphragmatic muscles are exercised and put to use. This activity strengthens those muscles and enables one to cough and clear the respiratory passages better, helping the prevention of bronchitis and pneumonia, and faster recovery from common ailments and flu.

All of the breathing passages are cleansed, all the alveoli are opened, and a fresh exchange of oxygen is delivered.

The mind becomes clearer and more relaxed. All the soft tissues and sphincter muscles also relax.

The physiology of sinus arrhythmia is that the heart rate varies during breathing cycles. It is well demonstrated that one can reduce the heart rate by 10- 20 beats per minute, by doing breathing exercises.

When taking rapid breaths of short duration for several times, a feeling of reinvigoration and energy boost is created. This is due to the effects of hyperventilation, leading to mild respiratory alkalosis and hypocalcemia.

Breathing exercises help in the treatment of bronchial asthma, COPD (Chronic Obstructive Pulmonary Disease), congestive heart failure, sinusitis, and allergic rhinitis.

Singers, musicians, swimmers, and other athletes practice breath-holding. It helps them to perform better. Athletes take a deep breath before they start a spurt of activity, such as swimming, running, or wrestling.

Breathing exercise helps to relax, pause, and helps with stress reduction, anxiety, and anger management. Muscle tension is relieved and slouching, sagging shoulders are straightened.

As a demonstration, please take a deep breath and count one to ten. A sigh of relief is made. You will notice that you automatically sit straight and your posture improves. Next, please feel the pulse on one wrist with the fingertips of the other hand. Now take a deep breath, hold it for as long as possible and then exhale. You will notice that your pulse becomes weaker and slower, showing that the heart rate and blood pressure are reduced during the maneuver.

Stretching Exercises: This part of Yoga gets a lot of attention in the media and in practice.

Various types of postures and positions are described, touting various special benefits. The bulk of what is being offered, as Yoga comprises of doing various postures. Let us not get into the details of these gymnastic postures that can be difficult and at times dangerous.

Stretching of various joints and ligaments and maintaining balances are practiced during Yoga exercises.

These exercises allow the flexibility of joints and tendons and improve muscle tone. They improve balancing ability thus reducing falls and slips and reducing the chance for injuries.

Reduction in back pain, arthritis, fatigue syndrome, pain syndrome, migraine, and headaches are noted. Sleeping and sex are reported to improve.

All athletes engage in a short period of stretching exercise before the actual commencement of their favorite sport. This allows them to perform better, with an energy boost and loosened muscles and joints.

Stretching can be an exercise by itself. It is done not only in Yoga but also in martial arts such as karate or Tae kwon do and in other gymnastics.

Passive static exercises of muscles are as good as active bursts of energy.

All exercises in any form are shown to control blood pressure, obesity, diabetes mellitus, and reduction in the incidence of heart attacks, strokes, and cancers. Yoga is an exercise by itself and all the various benefits of exercise apply to Yoga also.

Meditation: Meditation is the focused and controlled relaxation of the mind while maintaining a sharp awareness for short periods. It requires a certain amount of practice initially. It is not the same as taking a nap. It is a time out for the brain. It is a voluntarily achieved state between the conscious and subconscious mind.

The connection between mind and body is well documented, and several illnesses can be managed better with this understanding.

In our busy day-to-day life filled with pressure and stress, there is a need to pause and give a time out or rest for the brain. It gets refreshed and recharged.

It increases productivity, replenishes attention, solidifies memory power, and encourages creativity. It produces a state of relaxation, peace of mind, and a sense of tranquility.

Research with fMRI (Functional MRI) shows that meditation can increase blood flow to the hippocampus and frontal areas of the brain and increase gray matter.

EEG studies show increased alpha and theta activities in the frontal lobe.

Amygdala, which is an area that processes emotional stimuli, shows decreased activity during meditation. This allows one to face uncomfortable situations with calmness and enables one to tolerate pain with fewer medications.

The net result is stress reduction, increased empathy, happiness, and peacefulness. There is increased compliance with medical advice, reduction in drug addiction, and alcohol abuse. There is less impulsive behavior leading to gun violence, family quarrels, road rage, crimes, and accidents.

Meditation is very inexpensive and simple, and because it does not need any special equipment or set up. It can be done anywhere, anytime. It is up to each individual to effectively meditate by any method. It can be combined with religious protocols or prayer or it can be done in any way, as each one feels appropriate.

It helps with the management of anxiety disorders, diabetes, and hypertension, asthma, cancers, depression, and sleep disorders.

It reduces dementia and the need for pain medications. Management of pain-related conditions, as well as end of life issues, are made easier. It also increases the immune response of the body.

Meditation can be done in different ways. It can be focused 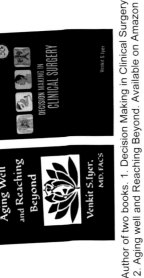 epeat a certain syllable or prayer or a focus on a certain image or idol. It can oat free. It can be combined with t of total silence. Retreat, solitude, at all cost), satyagraha (search for asam) can be variants of meditation. l to relax and staying away from the msara).

above three steps: The medical three parts: breathing exercises, meditation practices. They can be oarately.

itions and protocols with different ·ious benefits. There is much derstanding of what Yoga offers. ion or rules overseeing them. Many exercises and postures as seen in Yoga classes.

There is a mistaken opinion that this is the promotion of Hinduism, and Eastern philosophy or prehistoric recital of the outmoded Indian medical system of Ayurveda and such holistic protocols.

Very little training is required for anyone to become a yoga teacher. A recent article in the Wall Street Journal states that 15,000 yoga teachers are being certified each year in the US alone, after taking brief courses. There is much commercialization in yoga mats, clothes and apparel, and in yoga classes and yoga studios.

The medical benefits of yoga are now well accepted and proven. Breathing, stretching and meditation can be done at any time, anywhere, and at no expense. They bring in both mental and physical wellbeing.

It can be tailored to a personal level. However, group activities do bring in fun and opportunity for socialization. Doing yoga in naturally scenic settings allows one to enjoy nature as yoga does blend with the appreciation of nature.

The Nobel prize in 2009 was awarded for the discovery of the telomerase enzyme that keeps the DNA structure of chromosomes longer thus preventing the aging of cells. Yoga and meditation are shown to increase the telomerase enzyme level, thus indirectly suggesting that one can prolong life and slow the aging process.

There have been over 3000 articles of various research papers published about yoga in the last 10 years. The medical benefits of yoga are now recognized more than ever. Yoga by itself does not cure any illnesses, but it does work well as a complementary medical measure for better recovery from illnesses and to prevent illnesses related to lifestyle issues.

Over half of the medical problems and health care expenses can be traced to societal problems, lifestyle issues, and behavioral problems as their root cause. There is a lot of tension, anxiety, stress, and impulsive behavior, leading to family quarrels, gun violence, road rage, and criminal activities. We need to find methods that provide both mental and physical wellbeing. Yoga can be one such useful tool.

Chapter-5

STRESS REDUCTION AND SPIRITUALITY

Stress in life can reduce longevity. Blood pressure goes up, heart rate goes up and it increases the chance for heart attacks and strokes. Judgment becomes impaired, resulting in bad actions and consequences, such as road rage, road accidents, gun violence, and injuries. It also leads to obesity, alcohol use, or drug addiction. It affects sleep, and work performance. It can also affect marital life and social life and create family problems.

A new study authored in part by Moffitt Cancer Center in Tampa, Florida and Harvard T.H. Chan School of Public Health found that women who had experienced six or more symptoms of PTSD in their lifetime have double the risk of getting ovarian cancer, compared to women who never had that level of trauma. The study published in the journal of Cancer Research showed a link between PTSD and ovarian cancer. Stress hormones accelerate ovarian cancer.

What causes stress in life? Very often it is from family issues. Friction between expectations and reality. A fight between personalities. Difficulty in adjusting and adapting between two or more people. Disappointment waiting to be expressed. A desire to be dominant or a refusal to be subservient. A question of what one wants versus what is available. A feeling of being trapped with no escape. Feeling like being in a frightening dark corner due to self-inflicted wounds. The inability to meet other's expectations, being diminished in honor or respect. Difficulty expressing one's thoughts and needs because of constraints in society and family structure. Having a chocking sensation due to the dominant stature or pressure from elders or parents or peers. A failure in performance at school or the workplace. Or a physical disfigurement or complex that evolves and made to be an issue caused by the comments of others. Pressure builds up from childhood and becomes a behavior pattern. Also, sexual abuse in childhood leaves indelible marks on the person's personality and outlook. Demands to take care of children or the elderly with the necessity for work to make ends meet, along with demands at the workplace and associated transportation problems and household issues can create stress and a burden. Divorces, abortions, murders, and suicides are different manifestations.

Chronic and acute illnesses can cause stress. Painful conditions such as arthritis, back pain, cancer problems, degenerative conditions, hearing, and visual deficits, neurological problems such as paraplegia, paralysis, incontinence, need for frequent visits to doctors and hospitals, need for taking multiple medications are some of the examples that create stress for the individual as well as for the caregiver and family members.

Another cause of stress is work-related. Being overworked, verbal abuse, disinterest in the type of work you do, work that does not engage you or interest you, working below your level of skill, or working at a level above your ability. Also needing a better salary, financial concerns, not receiving promotions, or being passed over. Other concerns such as favoritism, nepotism, cronyism, needing time off or a vacation, needing to take care of children or family in times of necessity, an inability to participate in family functions, nagging, bullying, harassment of any sort, sleeplessness, traffic, communication issues, transportation issues, malpractice concerns, undue expectations from clients, patients or superiors, constant interruptions, the need for a high level of focus, multitasking, regular emergency actions, 24/7 involvement, media attention, social media, and public reports are all causes of anxiety and stress. Certain jobs such as that of a general surgeon or air traffic controller are known to be high-stress jobs by the nature of work involved.

Work-related stress is expensive for both employer and employee. According to a report from the Center for Disease Control and Prevention, in 2016, stress is the leading health problem in the workplace, affecting all levels of employees, leading to absenteeism, loss of productivity, and worker turnover. It also leads to depression, addictions, and obesity. Some of the measures found useful are regular work hours, adequate time off, greater autonomy, merit-based appreciation, and growth opportunities, and economic security.

Irrespective of the cause of stress, it takes a toll on the person's health. The individual is diminished in full capacity of performance and function. They withdraw from social and sporting activities. They tend to overeat and become obese. Lack of activity and obesity can lead to osteoporosis, hypertension, diabetes mellitus, stroke, and venous disorders. They also tend to be prone to develop behavioral problems, including commitment for suicides and homicides. The after-effects lead to more stress as a vicious cycle.

Some of the stress can be corrected by changes in daily routines. Avoid multitasking, over-scheduling, or tight scheduling; unnecessary deadlines and impossible time schedules are correctable. Take some time off during the day and make sure there is enough sleep. Other cases may need professional help or medications to calm the mind and to help with sleep. Put away the cell phone. Do not check it so frequently for messages and news. You do not have to answer phone calls or text messages instantly. Most of them can wait. Constant television watching and news cause more aggression and depression. Looking at a complex or stressful problem from another viewpoint or another's perspective may make it simpler to understand and solve.

This is a story of solving complex problems from a different person's view. A group of high IQ people went to lunch in a restaurant. They noticed that salt and pepper were in the opposite containers than marked on the cap. They launched into a high power discussion as to how they can switch the contents of the bottles without spilling and making a mess. They came to certain conclusions involving high tech intervention. The waitress came by to take orders. They decided to test her and told her that the salt and pepper were in opposite containers. She immediately apologized, leaned over, and switched the caps which had the marking of salt and pepper. Everyone was speechless. This story goes to show how a different perspective can solve a complex problem easily.

Spirituality is the ability to accept our place and duty in this cosmic world. It can be combined with religious beliefs or places of worship, which could be a church, mosque, or temple. However, to understand God, destiny, or fate, some people need to have the prop of religion, or a temple of worship, or a priestly figure. Yet others do not need such help. They do not need an idol or a place of worship. God is the same in all religions. It is we who end up using different names to address the same God. Prayer to God calms the mind, by agreeing to let a superior power to remain in charge and control the human lives.

Whether there is a God or not is a debate that has been ongoing ever since the origin of humanity. Most people believe in God in one form or another. There are of course atheists who believe God is a made-up story and hoax. Some agnostics agree to the presence of a supreme being but do not care for a name or a religion for recognition of God while wanting to live an auspicious life. It helps to leave the burden on destiny or God instead of having to take responsibility for oneself for the events that happen in one's life. It helps to pray in times of distress and misfortune, to find solace and comfort instead of feeling guilty and stressed. Certainly, most people will find peace and comfort in their last few days, by placing themselves in the hands of God.

The ability to forgive is one of the features of spirituality. Most of us have dark corners in our minds and we keep them as our secrets. Hatred and vengeance against certain individuals are not uncommon. Often it is out of some silly argument or inability to work together. We are just different people. For some individuals, it erupts as violence and homicides. For others, it is a matter of staying away from each other. But very few can forgive the so-called enemies. That takes a lot of mental maturity. If you can forgive the enemy before you die it will bring peace of mind. The best time to correct an error is immediately as it happens. Apologize as quickly as you can as soon as something bad happens so that it does not fester around and become a larger issue.

A bigger issue is to forgive oneself. None of us are completely good or completely bad. All of us are made of a mixture of both good and bad. It is a question of how strongly we express our feelings and how aggressively we take actions in response, and also how others perceive these actions. As we get older, the recollection of the errors and mistakes you made in your own life, parades through your mind during sleepless nights. If you count the mistakes you made on your own and feel sorry for the same, and if you can forgive yourself for the mistakes you made, and repent and make corrections and amends, it will give you more peace of mind before you die. Catholics and certain other denominations have a system of confession of one's sins, through the place of worship, seeking absolution.

Reasons why people make mistakes or unfair deeds are worth analyzing. Usually, it is for money, sex, or power and control. Fame, recognition, stature, self-ego, family achievements, and pride are some of the things that go with the above. History is full of wars, attacks, conspiracies, infidelities, murders, slavery, treason, and cutthroat competition. For the most part, the underlying emotion will be sex, money, control, or power. Power is very addictive; it is hard to let go of it. Controlling another human for your needs or your pleasure is intoxicating. All irrational and illegal actions will be justified one way or another. Then there are situations when one wants to take revenge for past events. To correct an old unfair action, a new unfair action is undertaken as a tit for tat. Sometimes mistakes are made out of sheer stupidity or ignorance, or wrong calculations. Sometimes it is done as an act of willful punishment.

Buddhist teachings say 'do no harm to others whether it be by deeds, words, or even by thoughts. Help others if you can. Accept the fact that the world is chaotic, and you cannot change it- so learn to live with it and adapt yourself.'

Chapter-6

LIFE AFTER RETIREMENT

Japanese people are known to work long hard hours, to the extent that they get depressed and become unhappy after retirement. A story goes like this: A retired Japanese person was sleeping at home during early morning hours. The teenage son asked his mother- "Who is this man sleeping in our house?" He had rarely seen his father, who would leave home before he woke up and usually came home after he was asleep. The Japanese have a higher rate of divorces and suicides after retirement. During the working years, they settle on a certain routine lifestyle. This gets disrupted leading to friction after retirement.

There are two reasons why many people are afraid to retire. First is the fear of boredom, and not knowing what to do with the newly found time. The second reason is financial insecurity. Will I need more money? Can I afford to retire? I need income to keep up with the expenses.

Financial security is a relatively easier problem to resolve if one had planned ahead of time. The habit of saving regularly should start at a young age, with money put into qualified retirement accounts. Unfortunately, over half of Americans do not save adequately and do not plan for retirement. Sometimes they make bad investments. Keep in mind that some of the expenses will be less in the retired life such as taking care of children; their education, and work-related expenses. Many people would have paid off home mortgages by this time.

However, new expenses such as health care needs may crop up.

New income will come in the form of social security benefits, and Medicare for health coverage. Mandatory withdrawal from the qualified retirement accounts after age 70.5 will add to the revenue. The estimate is that if one has no debts and no obligations for children, and if the mortgage is paid off, a couple can live on $50,000 per year for a lower-middle-class lifestyle after retirement. One would need $100,000 per year for an upper-middle-class life with some luxuries thrown in such as travels and vacation. If one has a nest egg of 2 million dollars invested carefully, this type of comfortable retirement would be possible.

Very wealthy people end up giving away a chunk of their wealth to charity. One can only spend so much money on personal needs. Many physician friends are already in the 90th percentile of income earners, but they still feel the need to make more. One should not be a workaholic whose goal is earning the last dollar in the world, because if you do not spend your money, someone else will. The smart thing is to plan for continuing the same lifestyle that you had during your working years for the post-retirement years as well.

The bigger problem that many people face is boredom and a lack of activities. This becomes very severe when one suddenly stops working from a full-fledged work schedule. If at all possible, one should avoid this "cold turkey" retirement, and start slowing down for a period of one or two years. It may not be possible for salaried employees, but self-employed people can certainly slow down, delegating the work to successors and working part-time.

When speaking about retired life, many people dream of lying on the beach with bikini-clad girls on both sides and uniformed bearers serving cocktails, or playing golf and having a beer in the lounge. That is what they see in the movies or read in the fiction, but in the real world, these things are rare. What is real, is that one will find plenty of time to do things that they'd put off during their working years. All the hidden talents and hobbies and items of interest can come out and be expressed.

The first thing one should do is to exercise regularly, now that you have all the free time in the world, to stay healthy. One can join a nearby gym which often will give a discount to seniors. I belong to a program called 'Silver Sneakers' through the health insurance plan. This allows me free membership to a qualified health club. Fortunately, we have a large YMCA in my neighborhood. It has tennis, swimming, a full gymnasium, yoga, Pilates, Zumba, and various group exercise programs. We take full advantage of this facility and go there around 9.00 AM and come back by 11.00 AM. Usually, I play two sets of doubles tennis at this time. This would have been impossible during my working days.

Learning a new skill or sport can be very engaging. I could never play golf during my working years since I would get called for emergencies any time, any day. After retirement, I joined a golf club in the neighborhood for just $50 a month under a plan called the Player Development Program. It allows one to practice in the range unlimited any day, any time, one golf clinic with a pro once a week, discounted cart fee, and free walking golf after 3.00 PM. I use it frequently as an evening walk while also enjoying the game. Over the past five years, I have become comfortable playing golf, and in the process, I have made many good friends.

This would be a good time to explore ideas one had in mind but were kept on the back burner due to busy schedules. It may be art, music, dancing, reading, writing, traveling, sculpture, painting, pottery making, carpentry, or gardening. Whatever the desire is, whatever the hobby is, now is the time to splurge on it with no inhibitions. You have the time, you have the money, and you are your own boss and you do not have to explain it to anyone. You are pursuing it for your personal enrichment. Retirement does not mean sitting on a couch all day. It means doing things that interest you.

I found that writing a book on clinical surgery was an enriching experience. I wrote the book titled "Decision Making in Clinical Surgery". Jaypee Medical Publishers in New Delhi, India published it. The book is a symptom-based approach to common surgical problems, written as a guide for medical students, interns, residents, and junior surgeons. Each of the chapters starts with a symptom or a complaint or what was noted as a problem during rounds. It describes the quickest way to make a diagnosis, perform the tests, and do the appropriate treatment. I wanted to transfer my years of experience and knowledge to benefit the younger surgeons.

Volunteering to help others or teach the younger generation is a satisfying experience. Medical missions in third world countries will open your eyes. For them, their very existence is a struggle with meager amounts of health care amenities, food, and shelter in these places. Poverty, pollution, corruption, and complacency are mind-boggling. Yet they put up with the misery and find satisfaction in what they have. The gratitude they express will bring tears to your eyes. Others may prefer to do their volunteering in local free clinics, hospitals, churches or temples, or other humanitarian projects.

I participated in various medical missions in third world countries, mostly teaching surgery to local area surgeons, junior surgeons, and medical students for the past five years. I went to India three years in a row, and also went to Tanzania, Cambodia, and the Philippines. The most rewarding experience for me was teaching the younger surgeons on techniques of various surgical procedures in the operating room. I also gave several lectures, some to general medical staff, and many times to medical students as formal classroom lectures.

Another good thing that happened in retired life was increased socialization with friends and family. Traveling used to be difficult and had to be scheduled to fit the work situations. Now I can travel anytime, any day, and even get senior discounts. We visit grandchildren more often than before. We play cards once a week with friends and we have dinner together afterward. This reduces stress in life. We have come to learn that life is "what it is" and we no longer try to conquer the world. Spirituality and prayers happen more often than before.

To come back to Japan, the best-selling book there in 2017 was a humorous book written by Aiko Sato, 95 years old, written in longhand "Age 90: What's so great about it". The best-selling book there in 2018 was "Life by Myself" depicting a 74-year-old woman's life. Another popular book "The Finished Person" describes the adventures of a retired person, falling for a younger person.

Retirement could be the best thing that could have happened to many people. They are less stressed and more at ease with themselves. There are no empires to conquer, fewer goals to meet except to stay healthy and independent as far as possible. Still, people may have different priorities. But there is no need to fear about retirement, and there is no need to keep working till the last day. There is life after retirement for those who want it.

Section-2 – Aging Well

Chapter -7

FATAL FALL

Last year I was shocked to hear about two of my friends, both are physicians in good health. One was brushing teeth in the bathroom when he tripped, fell over backward, and hit his head on the wall, and sustained a scalp laceration. He went to the emergency room, had the laceration sutured, and went back to his normal routine. Except for initial dizziness, there were no gross neurological deficits. He went to Europe on a preplanned two-week tour. He came back to town, went to work; drove around and everything seemed normal. A few days later he started having balance problems and dizziness. Feeling something was wrong, he went back to his physician and had an MRI scan of his head done and found there was a large subdural hematoma that was beginning to compress his brain. Immediately, he was seen by a neurosurgeon and had a craniotomy done and the hematoma was evacuated. He recovered well and has been normal since then. Everyone was amazed at the seriousness of the situation, how trivial it seemed in the beginning, and how lucky he was. This could have been a life-threatening situation from a simple slip and fall. Thanks to his lucky stars, he recovered.

Another friend was going for an evening walk in his neighborhood. He tripped and fell on the sidewalk, hitting his head on the concrete. He passed out, someone called 911 and he was taken to the emergency room in an unconscious state. The emergency scan showed a large subdural hematoma from this simple fall and he underwent an emergency craniotomy. Unfortunately, he remained comatose on the ventilator for three weeks, before he slowly recovered, and came home after one month in the hospital. Thank God, he is also normal now.

What I am saying is that these two, true events show that a simple fall can turn into something dangerous. Both of my friends could have died but made a miraculous recovery, yet many others are not so lucky. Particularly at risk are those who are taking blood thinner medications such as Coumadin, and those who have other comorbidities, for this could have ended up in death.

Many deaths that start with a fall that may initially look like a simple accident or slip. The elderly tend to break their bones or develop a brain injury resulting in hospitalization, surgery, and side effects that eventually snowball into the end of life.

According to an article published in the Tampa Bay Times in May 2018, that was reproduced from the Los Angeles Times article authored by Karen Kaplan, explained that a total of 29,688 Americans older than 65 years old died from falls and related problems in 2016. About one in four senior citizens sustained a serious fall each year prompting 3 million visits to emergency departments of hospitals across the country. Once every 19 minutes a senior citizen dies as a result of injuries sustained during a fall.

In the trauma bay of emergency rooms, the number of older people presenting with falls has surpassed younger people presenting with real trauma. A number of these falls are seemingly minor at home, yet present with serious problems such as fractures, chest injuries, and head injuries. Moreover, the fall and subsequent interventions can leave the person permanently disabled or can snowball into an end of life situation.

Conditions that make one more likely to fall include the following:

- An elderly state
- Toddlers
- Neurological deficits
- Lower body weakness
- Vitamin D deficiency
- Vision problems
- Hearing problems
- Medication effects
- Alcohol intake
- Drug abuse
- Improper footwear
- Balancing problems
- Attention distractions
- Careless attitude
- Hypoglycemia, diabetes mellitus

Mobile phones (cell phones) have caused a new set of problems such as:

- Listening to music or talking while walking or crossing roads, when warning sounds are cut off
- Texting while walking, climbing into public vehicles, or driving
- Playing games such as Pokemon while walking
- Taking pictures and selfies without watching for hazards
- Use of headphones or earplugs that cut off sounds of alert
- Watching videos while walking

Sporting injuries are another main reason for falls.

- They are higher with contact sports such as football, basketball, hockey, or soccer.
- Injuries are higher with skiing, snowboarding, rollerblading, horseback riding, parasailing, bungee

jumping, parachute jumping, where there is less chance of balancing and control by the individual.

Also, one should consider risk-reducing measures in the house such as:

- Living in a one-story house as compared to a two-story house with a staircase
- Even flooring throughout the house instead of having steps between rooms
- Rugs and mats should have flat and tight placements
- Keeping slippers and footwear away from doorsteps and the bottom of stairwells
- Installing grip bars in shower stalls, toilets, and other wet areas
- Having handrails on both sides of staircases
- Adequate lighting inside the house
- Keeping the floors with the maximum open and walking space instead of cluttering it with objects and furniture
- Keeping the house clean and tidy

Other measures of value are:

- Balancing exercises
- Having medical checkups to ensure safety
- Hospitals and nursing homes observe precautions and prevention of falls, which includes side rails for beds, restraints, sedation, and surveillance cameras, in extreme cases.

The CDC has a website for instructions and educational materials at cdc.gov/steadi (which stands for Stopping Elderly Accidents, Deaths, and Injuries). Another site for information is ncoa.org (National Council on Aging). Enter falls in the search box.

Chapter-8

GERIATRIC MEDICINE

Geriatrics is the care of the elderly as opposed to pediatrics, which is the care of the children. Similar to pediatric medicine, geriatric medicine has become a subspecialty of Internal medicine. With an increasing number of senior citizens in the country, it has become a necessary specialty. Special problems affecting older people, involving surgery, medical care, and long term care are addressed.

It is estimated that every day 10,000 people turn to age 65 in the United States. By the year 2030 one in five Americans will be over the age of 65. The need for health care of the elderly will be overwhelming. For example, in the trauma bay of major hospitals, the number of older people falling with resultant injuries has already surpassed younger people presenting with injuries. With advancing age, there is a general decline of all physiologic functions of the body. Any illness or surgery on the elderly can result in a higher level of morbidity or mortality, compared to the same insult to a younger person.

Heart and vascular disorders are the most common causes of death all across the board. Over 80% of such deaths are occurring in the elderly. This is not only due to heart attacks, but also due to congestive heart failure, irregular heartbeat, postoperative complications following surgery, and anesthesia. As we get older, the contractile power of the heart muscle declines, autonomic pathways of conduction are replaced with fat and fibrous tissue, and heart valves get deposited with calcium and cholesterol plaques. Peripheral arteries become narrow and irregular and blood pressure goes up, which in turn puts more pressure on the already diseased heart muscle.

Respiratory problems are more severe for the elderly. Ordinary upper respiratory infections, flu, or post-surgical recovery can become serious for them. The muscle strength to cough and bring up phlegm or a mucous plug is poor, for which as a result they develop pneumonia or a collapsed lung. Conditions such as COPD (chronic obstructive pulmonary disease), emphysema, chronic pulmonary fibrosis, sarcoidosis, and tuberculosis are common in older patients. They require antibiotics more often. Antibiotics have their side effects too. All the various breathing functions are weaker, and the lung itself has a lower elasticity. Blood clots develop more easily in the veins, which can travel to the lung and cause blockage of blood supply to the lung. All of these problems may require the use of artificial ventilator support or the use of a breathing machine. New sets of problems occur thereafter, requiring the prolonged usage of the ventilators.

Kidney function slowly deteriorates due to sclerosis of the glomeruli, disease of the arteries, metabolic problems, and immune-related issues. About 25% of the population over age 70 have moderate to severe kidney dysfunction. Kidney failure leads to further accumulation of waste material such as blood urea and creatinine and further metabolic problems that affect the entire body. The equilibrium of the internal milieu gets deranged. They may require dialysis or even kidney transplantation. These procedures can bring new problems and complications.

Diabetes mellitus is adult-onset type 2 diabetes. 20% of the adult population has adult-onset diabetes. The blood sugar remains high, leading to a whole set of medical problems, including neuropathy, retinopathy, vascular blockages, kidney problems, heart diseases, and wound problems. Control of blood sugar to an appropriate level is a long-term commitment, both by the patient as well as the health care providers.

Dementia, Alzheimer's disease, cognitive disorders, stroke, Parkinson's disease, depression, anxiety disorders, hearing loss, and visual loss are other sets of problems affecting the elderly. Not only do they require constant vigilance and attention, but they may also need medications, physiotherapy, speech therapy, and nursing care. The extent of disability may be different and variable. When they are unable to ambulate or become bedridden, they would need personal care and nutritional support as well. Studies show that the onset of dementia and Alzheimer's disease can be postponed by following the wellness measures described earlier, with proper diet, regular exercise, brain-stimulating activities, avoiding smoking, and socialization.

Cancers for some reason occur more often in the older population than younger ones. These require early detection and treatment. Such treatment may involve surgery, chemotherapy, radiation therapy, or immunotherapy. Different types of cancers carry different prognosis and treatment schedules. Heart attack, stroke, and cancers are the three most common causes of death.

Trauma is a frequent cause of death and disability. Elderly people have accidents due to hearing problems, vision problems, balancing problems, and slow reaction times. They tend to fall and break bones more easily due to osteoporosis and arthritis. They also tend to get head injuries and internal bleeding. Many of them may be taking anticoagulants (blood thinners) such as Coumadin.

Elder abuse and neglect is also a factor that leads to trauma. Elder abuse is a form of domestic violence. It is more pronounced than generally recognized and is vastly underreported. The patient is often unwilling or unable to complain. Physicians are ill-equipped to address this social problem. It can be in form of neglect, mistreatment, abandonment, sexual abuse, emotional abuse, financial embezzlement, physical torture, starvation, and verbal abuse. Some of the evidence of physical abuse of the elderly are: burn marks in unusual areas, bruises on difficult to reach areas such as the back, harsh arm grip marks around the upper arm, injuries to genitals, and fear of the caregiver by the person.

There have been several studies on elder abuse. Most of them take place at home, and the offender is a family member. However, the rate of abuse goes up in nursing homes. Even good-intentioned caregivers become overburdened after some time due to the demands of care. Some of the offenders are mentally deranged to start with. The elderly need to remain cognitively independent for as long as possible to protect themselves.

Vision and hearing impairment affects over two-thirds of the elderly. Correction of these deficits will significantly improve their lifestyle, reduce accidents, and increase longevity. Many of these impairments are correctable with surgery or appropriate devices. Common vision problems are cataract, glaucoma, retinopathy, macular degeneration, and a need for reading glasses. Eye floaters are tiny transparent specks and filaments or squiggly lines that float when looking forward and go away. This is an aging process. If they become severe, then they need surgery. Otherwise, they can be left alone. Common hearing problems are cerumen impaction, age-related hearing loss, and cochlear degeneration, and noise-related hearing loss.

Dental health deteriorates with advancing age. Gums recede, enamel wears out, and teeth decay. Periodontitis and gingivitis occur and gaps widen between teeth. Eventually, many teeth may fall out. There is a higher chance for oral and pharyngeal cancers occurring with advancing age especially for those who smoke and/or drink. Many elderly people have full or partial dentures associated with new sets of logistics.

Mental depression and chronic pain syndromes are more common in the elderly. Good numbers of chronic pains are related to back pain or arthritis-related disorders. In addition to pain medications, they need physical therapy, psychological support, and social support. Depression sets in along with loss of cognitive functions, loss of independence, and associated anxiety syndromes. In severe cases, they will require medications to alleviate the same, instead of brushing aside as emotional issues.

Based on studies conducted by John Hopkins Medical center and a survey conducted by the National Health and Aging Trends Study in 2015, it was noted that 25 million older Americans require daily help to function. This is excluding those in nursing homes, assisted living facilities, and other institutions. These are forgotten people by society and are dependent on family help or caregivers who receive little to no reimbursements. They need help with bathing, eating, getting dressed, transferring from bed, using toilets, and moving around inside the house. Many neglect themselves and suffer silently.

Chapter-9

PALLIATIVE CARE

Palliative care is a multidisciplinary approach to help individuals with life-limiting conditions, to improve quality of life rather than prolong life. It focuses on relieving pain, physical and mental strain, with the help of doctors, nurses, therapists, and other paramedical personnel.

The word palliation or palliative care is often used to interpret the purpose of a certain type of treatment or surgery, to describe that it is being done for symptom relief or for improving the success of other adjuvant therapies, but with no expectation of cure. For example, surgeons very often undertake procedures for "palliation" when a cure is not expected for cancer patients. Such surgical procedures include debulking a tumor for better effectiveness of chemotherapy (removing chunks of cancer but not all of it), doing bypass procedures without removing the tumor to overcome blockage of the lumen by the tumor, placing feeding tubes to maintain nutrition, or inserting a morphine pump for continuous infusion of pain medications.

Medications are prescribed for vomiting, dizziness, diarrhea, and insomnia and for the pain to alleviate those symptoms. In addition to cancers, they also treat chronic debilitating conditions such as chronic pulmonary disease, chronic heart disease, degenerative arthritis, and neurological problems, or HIV/AIDS. Palliative Care is an approved subspecialty of Internal Medicine with board certification for those interested in the field.

Palliative care is somewhat different from long-term care, end-of-life care, and hospice care, even though there may be some overlap between them. Palliative care does not automatically mean death is imminent. It can be provided in the hospital, nursing home, or at home. It is a planned and coordinated approach to make the patient more comfortable knowing well that the underlying health problem is not curable and the patient may live an undetermined length of time.

Symptom assessment is described in Edmonton Symptoms Assessment Scale (ESAS). The symptoms assessed are pain, vomiting, or nausea, depression, anxiety, appetite, sense of well-being, activity, drowsiness, and shortness of breath. Palliative care can be applied to children and the pediatric population as well as to adults or the elderly as needed.

Many individuals confuse Alternative Medicine or Complementary medicine with Palliative medicine. Such practices fall outside of the conventional modern medical advice unproven by scientific evidence. However, these practices are widely followed from time to time by a vast number of people, either out of blind belief, or due to the ineffectiveness of modern medicine, or they offer cheap and informal treatment. The so-called "placebo effect" is a well-known entity. Over some time, some of these techniques have received wider acceptance and are being integrated into modern medical practices. The following is a list of such practices, some are felt to be effective in palliative care, some are of questionable value, and health insurers do not reimburse any of them.

- Alternative Medical Systems: Ayurveda, Chinese medicine including acupuncture, Homeopathy, Unani, Siddha, Naturopathy, retreats,
- Meditation, mindfulness, Yoga, Tai- Chi, Prayer and mental healing, Herbal therapies, vitamin therapies, dietary supplements, massages, Ayurvedic massages, Reiki, magnetic therapy, and starvation and purging, holistic therapies, and laetrile treatment.

Chapter-10

LONG TERM CARE

Long-term care indicates that someone is assisting an incapacitated individual with medical care or personal care regularly, usually provided by a healthcare assistant. These issues may involve eating, bathing, ambulation, medication, physiotherapy, and nursing care. Such care can range from home health service to adult daycare, adult living facilities, and nursing homes.

When one reaches a certain age with diminished ability to be independent, or when a person sustains an injury or suffers from a life-threatening illness leaving the person debilitated, or when one needs help due to dementia or Alzheimer's disease, it becomes necessary to think about options of obtaining long term care.

There are graded levels of help available. A combined decision between the individual and family members along with the primary doctor can sort out the options. Also, one should take into consideration the financial and insurance status of the individual as to what is covered or what is affordable.

Options to consider are home assistance, home health nursing care, adult living facilities, nursing home care, and Hospice care. The choices depend upon the level of help needed, level of ambulation, mental capacity, disabilities, medical conditions, availability of one's family members, life expectancy, and financial status.

The simplest level is to get housekeeping assistance where an assistant or maid can come in to clean the house, cook meals, and do errands. Home health nursing care is useful for someone taking multiple medications, to check on the patients' medical state, wound care, or blood pressure. Getting help at home is the least expensive option. Another option is to move in with one of their children with some amount of privacy arrangements between parent and the children's family, in such a way that everyone has independence and help at the same time.

There are several low-cost ways of getting help at home. The Retired Senior Volunteer Program is a federally funded program to help less mobile senior citizens. "Meals on Wheels" delivers hot nutritious food once a day for a small fee. Many new website services and online food chains are now available that can provide fully cooked or partially cooked food as well as groceries delivered to the door. Online retailers like Amazon can reduce the need to go to department stores and supermarkets for ordinary supplies. Senior citizen centers are helpful sources of information, activities, and food.

Adult daycare centers can be a good supplement to home care. They provide daytime monitoring, meals, personal care, exercises, social companionship, and adult recreation activities. They can be half-day or a full day and can be one to five days a week. This will help working children to get time off without worrying about their parents. It could be helpful to call the National Adult Day Services Association at 877-745-1440 or check them out online at www.nadsa.org. Senior centers in your neighborhood are also good resources. Many of them provide social and recreational activities, education, and information. Meals may be available as well.

Independent living facilities are usually restricted to seniors, living in common grounds, who have common kitchens or limited cooking in the apartments and a variety of other living help. One step further is assisted living where the seniors are taken care of nearly completely with cooking, housekeeping, and medical care, but each person remains independent. Hospice care is for those having only six months or less to live.

A skilled nursing home is for those who are disabled and need around the clock personal care, nutritional support, and medical care, including physical therapy. Some of them are attached to hospitals in different formats. They can be a subacute care ward or step-down unit or it can be a skilled nursing facility inside the campus, but with separate admission records. They can also be in free-standing buildings independent of hospitals. One should check into the reputation of the facility and make a personal site visit before going into one of them.

Long-term care insurance policies are promoted and heavily advertised as a backup resource when the need comes. There are many pros and cons to consider before one decides to buy a policy. It is up to each individual to make an informed decision on this, after consulting his or her financial planners and family. In general, it benefits the insurance company more than the individual if one calculates the total premium paid and the total payout. It is a way of having peace of mind and a sense of security, but many will never use it or use only a portion of it. They are not financially good investments and can be expensive to start with. One is advised to read all the provisions, exemptions, riders, and conditions carefully before signing into one.

Medicare and Medicaid cover some portions of long-term care. Following hospitalization for major illness or surgery, short-term home health, physiotherapy, or skilled nursing home admission are covered. Usually, they are fully covered for the first 20 days, and partially for the next100 days. Hospice care is fully covered for six months. Medicaid rules vary from state to state and coverage is generally tied to the income level of the individual.

To get help in making decisions, and in choosing the most suitable options for your needs, one could discuss with your primary care physician and your family member. Word of mouth referrals from friends or acquaintances is also helpful.

Clergy, church, senior centers, county family agencies are other sources of information. The Agency on Aging is a government-funded program that you can reach at www.eldercare.gov or by calling 800-677-1116. One has to take into consideration specific medical needs, mental capacity, personal care needs, and financial obligations in choosing the right type of program.

Caregiving can be a difficult and expensive task. Because of the cost as well as the emotional levels, caregiving often falls on the shoulders of family members. It can lead to stress, interference with their own life and family, and affect their health also. It is estimated that 16 million unpaid and undocumented caregivers are taking care of someone in America. They need to find positive ways to reduce their stress, by talking about it with friends.

Chapter-11

HOSPICE CARE

Hospice is a Federal Government supported health and comfort care program for those who are terminally ill and have less than six months to live. Medicare picks up the tab irrespective of previous insurance status. President Reagan signed the Medicare Hospice bill in 1981. Since then there have been no changes to it.

The word Hospice is derived from the Latin 'Hospes', meaning guests and hosts. It was customary in the middle ages when pilgrims were given comfort or way-station during their journey on religious trips, from which they often never returned home. The modern-day hospice was first started in London in 1967. The first American hospice care was started in 1974 in New Haven, Connecticut. Today the word represents the philosophy or principles of end of life comfort measures rather than structures or buildings.

The National Hospice Organization describes hospice as a holistic, team-oriented program of care, which seeks to treat and comfort terminally ill patients and their families at home or home-like settings. The theme of hospice is comfort care with emotional and spiritual support.

To qualify for Hospice care, the primary care doctor must certify that the person is terminally ill with less than six months to live and refer the patient to a Hospice program and the patient must agree to comfort measures only with no further active therapy for the illness. Once it is established that the patient has exhausted all meaningful treatments and that there is no point in continuing maximum efforts to prolong life, it makes sense for the patients to seek pain-free comfort care in the last few weeks or months of their life and to die in peace and with dignity in their home. An example of such a situation would be someone who has advanced cancer which has spread all over their body and has already been treated with surgery, chemotherapy, and other modalities with no avail. In 2010 an estimated 1.58 million people in the USA received hospice care services.

Many people have the wrong impression that by accepting Hospice you have given up all hope, all treatments, and you are now embracing death. This is not true. Under hospice, one can continue to receive pain medications, nutrition, various comfort measures, and certain acute therapies. Differences of opinions between the patient, the hospice doctor, and the patient's own primary care physician can arise. Often this is due to miscommunication and misunderstandings. If a hospice patient falls and sustains a fracture or gets an acute infection, certainly they are admitted to the hospital and treated. They may even undergo surgery to provide palliation and reduce pain and suffering, but the hospice may not agree to intensive chemotherapy. Hospice provides reasonable care for palliation and management of terminal illness and related conditions.

Before entering into hospice care, most certainly one should make sure that all curable options have been considered in managing any illness. One should never give up hope. One should obtain second opinions when necessary, especially if the first opinion is disheartening. There can be mistakes or misinformation. The test results need to re-verified for accuracy and reliability. What is treatable at one hospital or medical center may be turned down as untreatable at another center and vice versa. One should review the pathology slides and make sure the diagnosis is confirmed as cancer. For the first time diagnosis of cancer, one must be very aggressive in treating it, with radical surgery, radiation, chemotherapy, or other newer modalities. We know the earlier we treat cancer, the better the chance there is of a cure. One should explore all avenues, do the maximum, and follow it up with necessary tests and additional treatment. What we are talking about here is the end stage of advanced cancer, where everything has been tried and it continues to advance. It is this stage where one has to be realistic. This is the stage when a consensus of opinions between all family members and doctors has been arrived at. That is the time to talk about palliative care and comfort measures. That is the time when it is rational to avoid more pain and suffering. That is the time to look towards salvation, peace, and religion.

The five "C's" for Hospice care are Communication, Collaboration, Compassionate care, Comfort, and Cultural care (Spirituality).

The most common location of Hospice care is the patient's residence. It can also be in a hospice in-patient facility or assisted living facility or nursing home, or in the hospital itself in designated areas. According to a report presented by the National Hospice and Palliative Care Organization in 2012, 66.4% received their care in their residence and 26.1% in a Hospice facility. An approved hospice program that is chosen by the patient takes over the entire care, which in turn provides a physician, nurse, and other health care workers as needed. They provide medications, medical equipment, hospital bed, nutritional support, and other personal care services. They will also provide physiotherapy, speech therapy, and emotional support as needed. They will not do housekeeping or cooking. They will continue to provide medical care for other co-existing medical conditions, provide pain medications, and monitor vital signs. The nurses render most of the care, with input from the hospice physician as well as the primary care physician if needed. It is possible to switch from one hospice program to another one if there is disagreement or dissatisfaction with the first one. They should also be able to help with some of the funeral plans and arrangements.

Once a hospice team has accepted the patient, they take over the entire care in consultation with the primary doctor or other treating doctors and family members. A team of health care experts arrives, which includes a hospice doctor, nurse, social worker, counselor, chaplain, home health aid, and trained volunteers.

The US Congress enacted the Medicare Hospice Benefit in 1986, and in 1993 it was established as a component of the healthcare government provisions. Medicare covers almost all of the hospice care. There is often a small copay. Medicaid and most private health insurances also cover hospice. Many of the Medicare advantage programs turn over the care to regular Medicare while under hospice. However, regular insurance will continue to cover unrelated medical problems. In fact, it is wiser to keep paying the premiums to Medicare A and B and to keep the Medicare advantage plan or other private insurance active, in case the hospice ends for some reason. It may be difficult to re-enroll at a time of dire need afterward. For example, one may be under hospice care for terminal cancer, but if there is a broken bone from a fall, that will be fixed under the Medicare or regular insurance. One can voluntarily decide to relinquish hospice and return to regular care at any time. Sometimes the person may live more than six months and go out of hospice and get back into it when the situation worsens at a later date.

There is at least one reported lawsuit between the Government and a hospice care center named AseraCare, (the US vs Aseracare) regarding the prediction of death within six months. The case involves 233 patients who were under hospice care between 2007 and 2009. The government hired a doctor to review those records to know if those patients had more than 6 months to live at the time certifications were filed. This doctor felt there were fraudulent claims. However, other doctors agreed that those patients had less than 6 months to live. There were disagreements between the jury and judge in the initial hearing, so it is under appeal with the 11th circuit court at the time of this writing. If fraud is proven then some of the doctors could face a penalty. The difficulty is to predict accurately whether one would die within six months or not. Such prediction of death can be more accurate in short-time segments of one day or one hour.

Hospice care and end of life palliative care have helped to reduce medical expenses significantly. About 30% of Medicare expenses are spent on the last year of life. Unnecessary ER visits and hospitalizations are reduced along with tests and treatments of minimal value. The proposal was made to cover End of life consultations, as a reimbursable fee for service to physicians under the Affordable Care Act. However, politicians made it a big scandal as payment for 'death panels' and were abandoned then. Now it has been reestablished as a reimbursable charge.

It is difficult for patients to give up hope and accept death. It is also difficult for doctors to say the situation is hopeless. They are taught to prolong life as much as possible using any recourse or technology. They will do any amount of interventions and tests and procedure, since accepting death is like accepting failure, but there comes a time for everyone to say enough is enough, and accepting hospice care is far superior to dying in the intensive care unit with tubes and needles all over the body.

We have heard of famous people who made common-sense decisions to die at home with friends and family in their bed and with comfort.

Senator John McCain was recently diagnosed to have brain cancer. It was a bad one called glioblastoma. He did undergo tests and initial treatments. On August 24th of 2018, he decided to stop all cancer treatment and entered hospice care. This was lauded as a wise decision, since the cancer was incurable, steadily growing, and would cause death within a short time.

Jackie Kennedy and Barbara Bush are two first ladies who come to my mind as well. They realized that the time had come and decided enough is enough. There was no crying, moaning, or lamenting. They celebrated their life and so did their families. Former first lady Barbara Busch stopped all medical treatments in the mid part of 2018. She had various medical problems, was bedridden, and was getting elderly. She had been admitted to hospitals several times before the decision. Having concluded that her death is imminent, she went into hospice care and had comfort measures only. As expected, shortly afterward she passed peacefully at her home with family and friends around her.

Both of them died within two days of the announced withdrawal of further medical treatments. Both their houses were open for all visitors and friends and families. Both had a dignified funeral with State and National honor. The publicity they received following such dignified deaths should give confidence to the average citizens to accept hospice care as the right thing for many people. Hospice care is not the same as giving up hope or expediting death. It is accepting realities and doing the best under the circumstances.

Hospice care addresses physical, emotional, medical, social, and spiritual needs for those facing life-limiting illnesses. They also provide counseling to family members and caregivers on issues such as cleaning the house and shopping. Hospice does not limit medical care, but it focuses on quality of life instead of trying to cure the incurables. A chaplain or religious priest is allowed to visit the person.

How do you find how hospice works for you? The easiest way is to ask your doctor or nurses or ask your friends who have used them in the past. One can go through Internet web searches also or can call 1-800-658-8898 for the National Hospice and Palliative Care Organization. For languages other than English the phone number is 1-877-658-8896. Once you select an organization, make sure you ask questions to your satisfaction before you sign up with them. Specifically, you want to know around the clock availability of health care workers in times of need and emergency and their track record in the community you live in.

Section-3 Getting things in order

Chapter 12

LIVING WILL

A Living Will is a legal document that describes one's preferences in treatment when faced with the end of life issues. It is also known as Advanced Directives on health care. All individuals, except minor children, are expected to have such a document prepared and made known to their immediate family members. The primary care physician should also know about it whenever possible. This will facilitate treatment and health care management in the desired fashion at the time of need especially when the patient is unable to verbalize the directives or opinions. A Living Will or Advance directives could cover items such as stopping life-prolonging undue treatments, recognizing the end of life issues, and managing persistent vegetative states. It can also address one's desire for organ donation or anatomical gift.

The most commonly sought out directive is whether to continue life support measures when one is in multiple organ failure and the prognosis appears to be bleak. Without such a clear directive, doctors in the hospital or intensive care unit will be obligated to keep the person alive and keep treating the person until natural death occurs. As we know, with advances in medical science, it is possible to provide such life support and keep the person alive for weeks and months.

Such a situation can cause a tremendous financial burden and the costs could run into several hundred thousand dollars. Moreover, it is a huge emotional drain on the immediate family, visiting the person in the intensive care unit daily and listening to the nurses and doctors, often asking you to sign numerous consents and permits, often explaining it in poorly understood medical vocabulary.

If we believe that death is an unavoidable eventuality, and if we believe that dying in dignity at home is better than dying in the intensive care unit with multiple drips and tubes in every orifice, then it is prudent for every person to set up a Living Will. All it says is that at a time when death appears to be imminent and when the medical prognosis is poor and when there is no meaningful hope of having a quality of life, and when the person is unable to make sound decisions due to the illness or health situation, the document now being made while in a sound state of mind and health should be used as a directive. It can clearly state that undue prolongation of life and meaningless life support should be avoided.

Such clear directives let the family members and doctors do the right thing without feeling guilt or prejudice. Otherwise, they may feel that they did not try everything in the time of illness to save the person. They may feel legally obligated to carry on with their routine work as per hospital protocols for fear of malpractice.

A Living Will clearly defines your wishes on individual items of care, as to what you permit and what you do not permit. For example, food and water are routinely administered to everyone, even after they have been disconnected from a breathing machine. Hence it is important to state that you do not wish to prolong life with food and water. This was an issue in several legal cases. Similarly, you can pick and choose procedures you agree to or disagree with. You may not want dialysis, but you may want a pacemaker inserted.

A Living Will is a legal document that must be executed by the person while in good mental health. Additionally, it is best to inform your directives to your next of kin, or spouse and your primary care doctor so that when an unexpected situation arises, they can get hold of the Living Will document and have it executed. Any attorney can prepare it as part of other legal documents for estate planning. Much of the information can also be obtained for free on web sites and can be copied. One does not necessarily require an attorney to prepare a Living Will for documenting advanced directives. Most hospitals have generic forms for Living Will execution. However, it must be in writing; a verbal understanding with the next of kin is not adequate.

There were no Living Wills up until 1960. It was a new concept then, and there was vigorous opposition to it from the Catholic churches and other rights to life organizations. It took years for the slow advancement of the concept. Due to rising health care costs, and the realization of meaningless prolongation of life and suffering at end of life, it has now become a very well accepted standard all across the country. The cases of Karen Ann Quinlan and Terry Schiavo (who were kept in vegetative states for over 15 years) and the likes received wide political and media attention.

A Living Will and a proxy or durable power of attorney must be executed by all adults and not just by old people. One may never know when and where destiny is going to play fowl. Accidents and head injuries can happen to anyone.

It is the responsibility of patients or families to inform the hospital and treating doctors about the presence of a Living Will. As a corollary, it is the responsibility of the hospital or doctor to ask the patient if they have a Living Will and document that information in the admission records. It may sound silly for minor illnesses, but one never knows when a catastrophe could occur. Therefore, it is highly important for those who have terminal illnesses, or advanced age.

A particular scenario is when the doctors write "Do Not Resuscitate" or a DNR order in the chart. This alerts all nurses and other health care professionals that no CPR (cardiopulmonary resuscitation) is to be called or conducted if the heart stops. Without such an order, they will call a "code" when all team members for the code rush in, do chest compressions, give an electrical shock, give medications, and insert a breathing tube or put on a ventilator, and so forth. Afterward, they are maintained on life support until a new decision is made.

A dilemma occurs when a person who is on a DNR order has to go for a procedure in the operating room. Some anesthesiologists insist on having the DNR order rescinded for the duration of surgery and reinstated immediately afterward. This is out of fear of malpractice and legal issues for doing something or not doing something in the operating room. They argue that surgery and anesthesia are by itself an invasion with resuscitation, and sometimes a cardiac arrest can happen even for a healthy person due to medication or ventilation issues. Still, there is no justification for doing a CPR (cardiopulmonary resuscitation) in the operating room on a patient with prior DNR orders and a Living Will. A good discussion with patient and family, empathy, and a realistic approach is needed instead of changing paperwork. These patients need the intervention despite their illness or advanced age for pain control or palliation or management of injuries. The patients as well as families very well understand and know that they are in a terminal state and death is imminent. They are just looking for less suffering and improved quality of life during the last days.

There are various ways to set up a Living Will. Advance directive forms are available on web sites of all state governments for free. Another site is Mydirectives.com, which has a cloud-based digital directive service to cover Living Will, health care proxy, and organ donation, which are legal in all states. Almost all the hospitals and surgery centers have a copy that one can sign on admission. All attorneys have formal documents for execution. One can also make one's own handwritten directives.

I remember a patient who presented with a very large abdominal aortic aneurysm. An aneurysm is the ballooning of a segment of the main artery in the body and given time they will continue to expand and eventually burst inside, resulting in a very high chance for death. When the aneurysm is 5 cm in size, it is recommended to have surgery to prevent such a catastrophe. This patient was 80 years old, had many medical problems and heart disease, and the aneurysm was 9 cm in size and ready to burst. We discussed the seriousness of the situation with the patient and family at length. The patient opted against any surgery since it carried a significant risk for him. He said that he had lived a good life, that he has no problems at this time, and when God wants to take him, he was ready, so this was documented, he was given medical treatment to keep him comfortable and to keep his blood pressure controlled. Three months later he presented to the emergency room brought in by ambulance in a state of shock and low blood pressure all indicating the aneurysm was rupturing. Tests confirmed the same. The same family who agreed to comfort measures three months ago wanted "everything" done to save his life including emergency surgery. The patient who was awake said he wants to do whatever his family wants so we were faced with the task of doing the complex surgery in an emergency setting with minimal preparations, which could have been done in an elective setting with the best preparations and precautions three months ago. At the insistence of the family, we did the surgery requiring several units of blood transfusion and several days of intensive care unit support. Eventually, he died ten days later. Afterward, I was talking to the family, as to why they decided to do the surgery at the last minute instead of doing it electively. Their answers were eye-opening. One said they did not want to share the burden of guilt of his death, another said that they feel good that everything possible was tried to save him, and another said that the insurance was meant for such catastrophic situations.

Chapter 13

DURABLE POWER OF ATTORNEY

This is a legal document that is prepared as a companion to the previous document of the Living Will. In this document one designates a certain individual or agent to act as the person's surrogate if and when a situation arises that renders the person unable to decide on his or her health care. It is also called a proxy for medical decisions or health care surrogate. The proxy must be over 18 years old and must be co-signed by two witnesses, one of whom should be unrelated to the person.

For example, one sustains a head injury in an automobile accident, requiring emergency surgery, and is in a comatose state for several days. The person named in the durable power of attorney can sign all the consents and permits, which are usually required by the hospitals. If there were no such documents, they usually go by the order of next of kin protocol. First in line would be spouse, then children of bloodline, then brothers or sisters. If there were no one available, then they would look for a legal guardian. If none were noted, then they would ask the risk management department to obtain a court-appointed legal guardian.

Sometimes we have witnessed situations where the spouse is divorced or disinterested or demented. Children may be in far off cities. It is good to have someone you trust and dependable to take care of your affairs.

It is important once again to have the document prepared by an attorney, and have your desires communicated with the named person in detail. This can avoid many hurdles in the unforeseen circumstances and emergencies as to actual care as well as the end of life issues.

Similar to a Living Will, this document was a new concept in the '80s. California passed the first law allowing durable power of attorney in 1983 and it was named the Medical Proxy Law. It makes sense since any individual may become unable to express his or her wishes. Now it is allowed as a valid legal document in all the states in the country.

Another use of durable power of attorney is to execute it to handle financial matters when one is unable to or incapacitated to handle them on one's own. The person who is entrusted to be the POA should be at least 18 years old, or a recognized financial institution. Two witnesses should sign them and at least one should be an outsider from being a blood relative.

Chapter 14

OTHER FINANCIAL DOCUMENTS

There are several documents pertaining to one's financial affairs that can be executed to ensure that assets are properly distributed according to one's desires, and the core of the money is protected as much as possible from creditors, Government, taxation, lawyers, and the court system. Once again, they are set up legally with help of attorneys, with appropriate planning, due thought process, and discussions with family, beneficiaries, lawyers, and financial planners.

Wills: This document describes how one wants the assets to be distributed after the demise of the person. If there is no will at the time of death, the court appoints a lawyer to probate the assets. The inheritors will have to go through more expensive and prolonged probate to get the assets distributed. Jointly owned properties and accounts held "in entirety" with a spouse would be exempted. Generally speaking, the process is much simpler with an executed will. Unmarried couples will not qualify for any benefits, even if they have been living together for years. A will is the only way to recognize and reward friends, servants, maids, charitable organizations, and religious institutions.

Trusts: There are several types of trusts. In general, they allow certain assets to be held in a separate entity, created with a certain goal and objective in mind. It can be revocable or irrevocable. There can be many stipulations in the trust, as to how and when the benefits are distributed, how it gets dissolved, how long it runs, who are the trustees and successor trustees. A generation-skipping trust can stipulate the benefits that run through two or three generations, instead of all the distributions going to the first generation. Trusts are useful vehicles for those with large assets since these vehicles can function as independent entities. Properties can be transferred to the beneficiaries directly without going through probate.

Estate planning: This protocol helps to minimize the tax burden on the estate left for an inheritance so that the inheritors get to keep more of the assets. This is based on estate tax laws, which have varied from time to time. They were also called the death tax in the common language. This is done through a variety of financial decisions, and not by a single document. One should consult a financial planner. The goal is to pay as little death tax as possible.

Charitable Foundations: This is for people who have very large assets. One can spend only a certain amount of money on luxuries and expenses for personal needs. Very rich people will have to decide what to do with the large sum of wealth they have accumulated over their lifetime. One good way is to find a vehicle that will carry their legacy that will help humanity at large. Charitable foundations can be set up that will help education, health care, humanitarian issues, and so forth. They can be set up in such a way that they encourage research, development, and inventions. Many famous individuals have their foundations for many years that are helping hundreds of less fortunate people. It allows them to know how their fortune will be spent when they are alive. Their philanthropy gets full credit and respect.

Life insurance: This is for risk protection of the beneficiaries, usually for a spouse or children. The benefits are not for the individual. It has no value for the person purchasing the insurance. However, it can be a good asset protection tool, if planned carefully. For example, if a whole life insurance policy is purchased for a large amount with cash payment, it is not yours anymore and it is away from the creditors. The policy can be made "second to die" which can almost double the face value. "Second to die" is an arrangement with the insurance company where the payment is delayed until both the owner and spouse die. The policy can then be transferred to an irrevocable trust, held for the benefits of children or grandchildren.

One other option to consider is to take out the cash value of a whole life insurance policy. The advantage is that the extra cash is immediately available for expenses of oneself. At old age, the children are probably grown up and independent and not in need of support. The policy was probably taken at a time when they were young. The disadvantage is that the benefits will be reduced, and beneficiaries may change, and one may have to pay capital gains tax. It may make the person ineligible for Medicaid if that is being used for nursing home care or terminal care. It is best to consult with a financial adviser in these situations.

Many of these documents come into effect after your death and get executed based on the directions you have set up. However, there is a scenario where you are still alive but unable to make decisions on your own. It can be a mental disorder such as Alzheimer's disease or dementia or a physical disorder such as stroke or head injury. You could be kept alive for an indefinite period. For these situations, you need to set up a durable power of attorney for financial matters. If no specific directives are made, usually your spouse or legal next of kin will handle it. The worst scenario is when an outsider such as a homemaker or a court-appointed guardian, makes these decisions.

Fraud and abuse: Older people without family support are targets for various types of fraud, abuse, and scams. At times it is their extended family members, neighbors, housekeepers, or caretakers doing the misdemeanors. Their main goal is to skim your money. Many stories are heard such as an 18-year-old girl marrying a 90-year-old man or keeping the elder person confined to the house for social security checks, or making them sign authorizations for expenditures that are extravagant, and so forth. Con artists know that the elderly are vulnerable physically, emotionally, and mentally. Telemarketers, door to door scam artists, and online fraud artists can easily blackmail and skim the vulnerable and incapacitated ones.

One methodology the con artists use is in the pretense of house maintenance or repairs. Since the elderly cannot do some of these repairs by themselves, they end up calling for assistance. The con artists makeup issues and pry large sums of money. They promise quick work at a low charge and then end up ballooning the costs for unwanted or fake work. Make sure that a written estimate is provided first, and a written contract of work is provided, and receipts are given in writing for all payments. Another common trap is an offer of prizes or cash if one signs up for something on the computer via the Internet. The computer is hacked immediately, and all personal information including bank accounts and credit card information is stolen. Telephone calls can be scams: either by promising something or threating to take any action unless immediate payment is made. Many phone scams are known to occur, but keep in mind that Income tax services, social security offices, police departments, or immigration officers never make phone calls. Either they present themselves at the door with the badges or send written letters.

Chapter 15

ORGAN DONATION AND TRANSPLANTATION

One hundred years ago there was no science or awareness of organ transplantation. Today over 25,000 such surgeries are done annually and over 100,000 patients are waiting for an organ in the United States alone. This is one of the miracles of modern medicine. Alexis Carrel a French surgeon developed a technique to suture blood vessels together, and forty years later drugs to reduce the rejection of transplanted tissues were developed. These were the milestones in the science of transplantation, discovering the technical and biological or immunological basis of organ transplantation. With experience and practice, organ transplantation has become routine in many centers. The first successful kidney transplantation was done in 1954 between identical twins.

Now kidney transplantation is a very common and standard procedure all across the globe. Organs used to be taken from brain dead people. Now they are also taken from living donors, when appropriate. Organ transplantation of liver, pancreas, intestines, and islet cells for insulin production; skin, face, limbs, bones, cornea, heart, and lungs are being done regularly with varying success. Part of the liver can be transplanted from a living donor or a whole liver can be transplanted from a cadaveric donor.

Those who wish to donate their organs after death can convey their wishes in various ways. A car license renewal is one such occasion. One can explain in their Living Will or durable power of attorney or via their regular will as added clauses. It can be informed to the hospitals upon admission. Organ donation agencies such as Life Link are willing to sign up and register donors. Doctors will decide if the person is suited to donate the organs since not all individuals are fit for organ donation. Ideally, they should be young healthy individuals with no diseases of any kind. Particularly they should not have cancers, or infectious conditions such as HIV/ AIDS, tuberculosis, and cirrhosis of the liver. Brain dead individuals otherwise healthy, such as gunshot victims or automobile accident victims, with other body organs still working are suitable for donation. A new development is now that HIV/AIDS and Hepatitis C are no longer a contraindication for organ donation since these diseases can be cured. Recipients are willing to take these organs instead of waiting indefinitely for a better organ.

Usually, the hospital notifies the agency once such a candidate is admitted and if the family or power of attorney agrees to the donation. Once the person is certified dead by the doctors, then the organ harvesting team arrives and removes all organs intact as quickly as possible and transfers the organs to waiting hospitals matching them with recipients. Modern computerization, database, communication systems, and transportation methods, the readiness of hospitals, and the availability of operating rooms are all factors that facilitate a smooth functioning system.

It is truly an appreciable and noble gesture that one would agree to have one's organs donated in case of death. Many people do not agree with donations due to religious reasons, fear, or personal preferences. However, it is to be noted that the organs are life-saving for the recipients, and the donor cells are living in the new body. This is to be seen as one form of immortality. Death may have taken parts of your body but other parts are living elsewhere.

Surgeons who are involved in procuring organs and transplanting them in others are called transplant surgeons. Marked progress was made in the 50s and 60s in the successful transplantation of organs with better immune suppression therapies and better techniques. Yet one single problem that has been felt all along even today is the availability of good donors.

One of the handicaps had been the suitability of matching the tests between the donor and recipient. To overcome this problem, a chain transplant system has been developed. Let us say patient A needed a kidney from patient B who was an otherwise suitable living donor, except for the matching tests. Then through the registry, they locate person C who needs the kidney who matches the kidney from person B. However, person D who was willing to donate patient C is found matching to give it to patient A. Thus, A gets the kidney from D, and C gets it from B. This type of chain living donor-recipient model can include three of four sets of people, all coordinated through donor registries, all having surgery at the same time.

The definition of death requires the heart to stop beating on its own. By then many of the organs have become unusable due to lack of oxygen in the tissues. Traditional ethical principles guiding organ donation/harvesting are referred to as the "Dead Donor Rule". Vital organs may not be removed before a person is declared dead and procurement of the organs may not be the cause of death of the person. This is to assure that the individual's interests and life is protected before the recipient's interests.

The field changed when the definition of brain death was accepted as a measure of death, but this required legislative changes. Such legal victory allowed Dr. Christian Bernard in 1967 to do the first heart transplantation in South Africa. Kansas was the first state in the US to allow the brain death concept and other states have followed. This single change has allowed numerous transplant surgeries to be done successfully, especially for heart transplant cases.

However, brain death is a difficult diagnosis and can be confused with several terminologies such as coma, permanent vegetative state, unconscious state, minimally conscious state, or loss of higher brain function with retained brain stem function. To make matters worse one can flip from a borderline zone to another and flip back again. Some individuals with no brain function may retain some occasional uncontrolled reflex motions, making one believe that they are on the path to recovery. Even trained doctors have been fooled in their predictions and the literature is full of anecdotal cases where a dead person has woken up.

Countries of Netherland, Belgium, Luxemburg, and Canada allow voluntary euthanasia legally where the physician is allowed to administer the lethal medication at the request of the patient. This has opened up some room for discussion on organ donation from these individuals. Many of these patients die at home and may have terminal cancers and thus are unsuitable for organ donation. However, some others can make prior arrangements to be admitted to the hospital ICU for the euthanasia to be immediately followed by organ harvesting. Even then ethical and legal questions have to be addressed. One problem is that an interval of 2 to 10 minutes is required before a full determination of death is made by which time many organs have blood clots and ischemia. One solution considered is to take them to the operating room and give them deep anesthesia and ventilation while the heartbeat is stopped with medications. The absence of pulse and heartbeat is confirmed while maintaining oxygenation, and quick harvesting of organs is done on the table.

The Canadian Supreme Court recently (2015) decriminalized medical assistance for dying in patients suffering from grievous and irremediable illnesses. Canadian legislature passed the legislature in the following year (2016), permitting physicians to hasten death by physician-assisted suicide. These rulings have created new pathways for organ donation in that country. (New England Journal of Medicine-Sept. 6, 2018- vol379- Page 909-91) In order to harvest the best suitable organs, they must be removed while the heart is still beating. This requires some amount of planning with the recipient waiting and donor willing to be undergoing death by organ removal under anesthesia.

In China, those who are to undergo execution for crimes are considered as candidates for organ donation. They are allowed to donate their organs in this way.

Chapter 16

FUNERAL ARRANGEMENTS

The funeral is the final farewell of the deceased person and for the disposition of the dead body. Mourning is associated with this process, as is respect for the dead person and their family, expressions of sympathy and support, participation in the bereavement, a celebration of life, and eulogy. Religious and community customs and cultural preferences are observed in various rituals, arrangements, and observations. Prayer for salvation for the soul is part of it.

Reaction to hearing news of the death of a dear one can be unpredictable. The bereavement process can vary from person to person. Generally speaking, the grief period can be in three phases. The first phase is one of disbelief, shock and numbness, and panic. There is a sense of denial, crying, loss of time, and place. During the second phase, there is a sense of acceptance, and reality sets in. They make funeral arrangements, viewing or wake and contact the funeral home and attorneys and financial advisers. The third phase comes later when they start reconnecting with the world, and getting back to the usual routine of work or hobbies and engage in social activities, with memories of the past.

Dr. Elisabeth Kubler- Ross in1969 described the five phases of grief. At first, there is denial- it cannot be true. Are you sure about it? Then there is anger- how did this happen, what went wrong? Then there is a phase of bargaining- what if, what can be done now? Then depression sets in- crying and mourning.

Finally, there is a phase of acceptance. Life goes on and adjustment occurs.

It is not uncommon to witness a period of confusion, stress, and a sense of urgency, immediately after confirmation of the death of a dear one. Many tasks have to be completed in rapid sequence and in an organized manner. For the spouse and immediate family member, it could be too much and numbing. It would be ideal to have a family member or a close friend to take over the function of the coordinator or CEO for a short period since the next 48hrs is going to be rapid and busy.

The first action is to make sure that a doctor is going to issue a death certificate. This may sound simple and automatic when a person dies in the hospital. If the person dies at home it would be better to have the family physician or hospice physician to come to the house and do the certification. The general tendency is to call 911 and have the paramedics come to the house. This would be a wrong step. Since they cannot certify death, they would end up taking the dead body to the emergency room to be certified by the emergency room doctor. Then the body will have to be shifted to the hospital morgue and they have to get the coroner's permission to release the body. It becomes much more costly, with the ambulance fee, emergency room fee, and hospital fee.

The next step is to prepare the body for transport to a funeral home and prepare for any protocols before that. Some families like to bathe and clothe the body, after removing all the tubes and needles. Nurses may be able to assist in this. Permission from the coroner is obtained if necessary. The funeral home is notified if one has already been selected. Some families arrange to hold a viewing at the home, some at the funeral home. Some may want prayer or religious service rendered privately at home.

A funeral home is to be entrusted with the final ceremonies. This is decided based on location, religious preferences, cost, type of burial, and family decisions. Most of the time it is a funeral home in the neighborhood. However, we know of many situations when the body is transported to a distant hometown or even to a different country of origin.

In general, for most people in modern times, the choice is between cremation and burial. Hindus prefer cremation. In the past, they created a large pyre using wood and other combustible products. This type of cremation, burning the body in open fire is practiced even today in rural areas. However, in the cities, western-style crematoriums have sprung up, where the body is turned into ashes within a short time in high-temperature furnaces. After the cremation, the ashes are placed in an urn and the family takes it home to disperse it in the waters or grounds that had been favored by the deceased individual.

Christians, Muslims, and Jewish people, in general, prefer burial. Yet many of them also opt for cremation nowadays. Burial is done in a cemetery connected to the church or mosque. The body with clothing and trappings are laid inside a casket and is lowered into the pit dug on the designated spot and covered back with the earth. A memorial slab or structure is erected, with a nameplate carrying the name and dates of birth and death.

More and more Americans are now preferring cremation instead of burial. The land is becoming scarce, and people are becoming more sensitive to environmental aspects. 99.9% of Japanese cremate. Jewish people are now opting for cremation commonly. Even Catholics are allowed to cremate as long as they do not separate and scatter the ashes, but it must be laid to rest in total in the cemetery according to a directive from the Vatican in 2016. The costs are three times more for burial as opposed to cremation. Most cities in the USA will pay for cremating an unclaimed body or for those in extreme poverty, but they will not pay for burial because of the cost. Many new steps are being taken to scatter the ashes. The time-honored method is to let the ashes float in the deep waters. Drones are used to spread them over land, special memory jars with ornamental carving are made to safe keep them on the house, and one firm even sends it to space.

Many individuals do make certain plans ahead of time for their funeral, even though this may sound funny. One can certainly make their preferences known to their immediate loved ones. Modern cremation has become clean, effortless, and is receiving increasing preference. An individual can also pick a certain funeral home or casket ahead of time, prepare their life story to facilitate the obituary, and even plan a funeral service, with the type of music, name of the invitees, and name of the priest. For example, Senator McCain made it clear that he did not want President Donald Trump to attend his funeral service.

All friends and family need to be notified of the death immediately by e-mail, text message, or phone calls or letters. A date and time for wake or viewing, service by a priest, or celebration of life with speeches by friends or family has to be arranged, followed by burial or cremation for which a date and time has to be fixed. A hall, microphone, flowers, photographs, PowerPoint projections, refreshments, guest book, music, or prayer chanting are all matters of importance. An obituary has to be written and provided to the news media and an announcement of death or celebration of life has to be notified to any organizations, institutions, or social and professional entities that the person belonged. Jewish people and Hindus arrange a celebration on the 13th day after the period of mourning when the soul is liberated to the heavens.

Depending upon the religious beliefs, personal preferences, and financial state of the family many different arrangements are possible. Added to this are the local and community situations and legal protocols if any. The popularity of the individual, political status, military status, fame, and reputation are additional factors.

In the Democratic Republic of Congo, it is the belief that there must be formal grieving with crying for at least one week after the death of a person, failing which the soul will get very angry and punish the family. Even though the body is no longer alive, the soul is lingering on and watching the reaction of the family. If you do not cry vigorously and mourn formally the angry ancestors will disrupt the progeny. Moreover, it is shameful by social standards that the family does not cry at their loved one's funeral. The requirement is so mandatory that many families hire professional mourners to cry. It costs nearly $1,500/, plus food and expenses, to hire ten women to cry and mourn for a week. They do a good job in return.

In the ancient days, Egyptians embalmed the dead body and made them into mummies, and kept them inside the pyramids or similar tombstones. The famous pyramids of Egypt are just tombstones. Some of the ancient priests, bishops, and cardinals were buried inside some of the famous cathedrals or churches. Some of the famous monuments and tourist spots are monuments built over tombstones. Examples are the Taj Mahal and Humayun's tomb in India, and the pyramids in Egypt. Leaders of nations or founders of nations are recognized with national mausoleums or memorial gardens, such as Raj Ghat for Mahatma Gandhi in India or Hochiminh Memorial in Vietnam. Very formal protocols or ceremonies are observed, and visiting dignitaries usually place a wreath in respect.

After the ceremonies are completed and the dust has settled, it is time to look into all legal and financial matters. Life insurance companies are notified of the death of the owner and the beneficiaries have to make their claim. Accountants or lawyers need to be contacted to enact the will and set the probate in motion. Real estate properties jointly owned need their deeds corrected. LLCs or corporations need a new chairman or directors nominated. Joint accounts need a change of ownership to solo names by notifying banks or brokerage firms. Inheritances to family need to be set in motion. Tax laws and legal protocols need to be looked into. Donation of a person's belongings such as durable medical equipment, clothes, shoes, medications, and such items that are of no use has to be channeled into charitable organizations. Items of memorabilia such as certificates, diplomas, personal jewelry, photographs, awards need to be gathered for safekeeping.

Thoughts are given for establishing memorial funds, endowments, scholarships, or charitable organizations in the name of the departed person, depending upon the cause and financial state. Eventually, the painful journey of illness, bereavement, and sadness has to end. New social activities or interests have to be established - life has to go on. That is the law of nature- the cycle has to go on.

Funeral rituals are as old as mankind in history. Evidence of funeral rites and protocols can be observed in most ancient civilizations. Egyptians mummified them and paced inside the pyramids. Greeks, Romans, and Indians preferred a funeral pyre with wood and other combustible items. Islamic, Jewish, and Christians buried the body kept inside a casket. Ancient Peruvians placed the dead body in a cave, and when decomposed, took the skeletons for memory gardens in their residence. Zoroastrians placed the body on a high open place to allow vultures to eat it, as a way of recycling the body and feeding other living creatures. The customs were dependent on the individual's culture, community, and religious beliefs. Many of them bathed the body and covered it with clean white clothes. Hindus had the body placed with their feet facing south, while the Islamic had the body facing Mecca.

In modern-day customs in the USA and Canada has become more secular with three events, namely visitation or viewing, funeral, and celebration of life or memorial service. All of these are coordinated through the funeral home and a priest, along with family and friends.

During the visitation or viewing, the body is placed in a casket, covered with the best clothes or the favorite clothes of the deceased, jewelry is placed, and the place is decorated with flowers, and soft music or religious chanting is played in the background. The spouse and immediate family sit in the front for guests to walk by and express condolences. There are no speeches or services. A guest book is placed at the entrance of the hall for guests to write their remarks. Photographs, medals, certificates, and diplomas are displayed, and milestone events in life are presented. Soft drinks or water is kept available. Bodies of famous persons and politicians may have the viewing extended for two or three days, whereas most ordinary people limit this process to three or four hours only.

The second phase is the actual funeral itself. Often this is kept as a private event, attended by only family and close friends. A priest is present to conduct a service based on religious preferences. The rituals according to customs may vary from two to four hours. Most pray for the soul to find solace and to reach heaven. After the service is over, the actual disposition of the body is performed. At this time all jewelry is removed and other metals are removed. Some remove pacemakers and such objects under the skin to allow cremation. The choice of final disposition is between cremation and burial.

The final phase is a memorial service or celebration of life. Many people conduct this same day evening of the funeral or on the next day. Jewish and Hindus have a mourning period of 12 days. On the 13th day, they celebrate the release of the soul to heaven. Formal religious prayers are sung, followed by eulogy or speeches by friends and family. Soft music or religious songs are played in between. Photographs and medals and diplomas are displayed in the lobby with a guest book for visitors to sign in. Milestone events of life may be presented by a PowerPoint presentation. Afterward, sumptuous food and soft drinks are served. There is no crying or mourning at this time. It is to bless the soul. It is a celebration of the soul.

Section-4- Death

Chapter 17

WHAT IS DEATH

Death is the cessation of all biological features of life for the entire body. The body shuts down completely and permanently. All bodily functions cease to exist. No voluntary or involuntary reactions remain. The body becomes just another inert material similar to a log of wood. Left alone, it decays and decomposes due to bacterial reactions, and emits a foul odor similar to a dead bird or rat in your attic. All the soft tissues slowly evaporate, leaving the skeletal bones in place for years and years.

A part of the body can die but the person can still be alive. For example, a toe can become gangrenous. At that point, the toe has no life. The toe has no sensation, no movement, no bleeding. The toe can shrivel off and remain as an appendage. In the current medical world, the doctor will recommend the toe be amputated. Later the doctor will do tests to see why it became gangrenous, and do surgery to protect the rest of the body or limb from the spread of the gangrene. Despite the gangrenous toe having died the rest of the body lives and functions well.

We can extend this analogy to many other parts of the body. For example, the whole leg or arm can be gangrenous and they can be amputated. The person can be fitted with an artificial limb later on and can go on functioning with some disabilities. An internal organ can be completely non-functioning or even totally removed by surgery and the person can live well. Sometimes the doctor recommends removing an internal organ to save the life and avoid the death of the whole body. The loss of such an organ never causes any future problems. Examples are when an appendix is removed when it is inflamed with appendicitis, or when a gallbladder is removed when it has stones in it or it is inflamed.

Organs that can be removed safely with minimal side effects include the spleen, parts of intestines, appendix, gallbladder, breasts, testes, varicose veins, and hair. Some of the organs are paired and one of the pairs can be removed and the other can function to keep the body alive. We can live normal with only one kidney or one lung, one breast or one testis. Parts of certain organs such as the liver, skin, lung, stomach, and intestines can be removed and the rest of the organ can regenerate and keep the body alive. Therefore, it is obvious that the body can still be alive and function well even if a certain organ is totally or partially removed. The question comes up as to how many of the organs can be removed before the entire body perishes. In other words how much insult it can take before the entire system collapses.

In the intensive care units of hospitals, people can be kept alive and well even if one or two organ systems have failed. For example, if someone has only heart failure or pneumonia, or kidney failure they can be treated and kept well. When more than three organ systems fail, then the chances of survival become low. The higher the number of simultaneous organ failures, the higher the chances of mortality.

Three main organ systems that keep the entire body working are related to the heart which sends blood to all tissues, the lungs which keep the blood oxygenated, and the brain that keeps the neurological functions. Therefore, when the doctors want to declare someone dead, they look to see if the heart, lungs, and brain are still functioning or not. Only when all three of these organs have stopped working for sure, is when they declare the person is dead.

If the heart alone stops, the blood can be pumped with an artificial assist, if the lung alone stops the person can be kept on a breathing machine, and the brain alone stops, the person can be kept alive in a comatose state. Sometimes all these three organs are working only partially because of disease or injury, but the person is still living in a disabled state.

There are situations when it is difficult even for doctors to certify whether a person is dead or not. This is because the individual has been kept alive for a certain length of time by various life support measures. They will have to stop these life support measures and give it some time to see if the body will live by itself or not. This becomes a very delicate legal and moral question in today's world. No one wants to be the one to "pull the plug" as they say in the hospitals.

This is where a consensus opinion and decision is needed. The family has to agree, all the doctors who are involved should agree that the situation is hopeless and there is no chance for a meaningful recovery, the hospital administration and risk management team should also verify, and all agreements have to be documented in the chart. At least two currently treating doctors should certify that stopping life support is recommended. Still, a question lingers as to what steps are to be taken first, what steps are to be continued, and for how long.

When I look back on my medical training, I had 14 years of medical training, between medical school, internship, residency, and further postgraduate training. During all these periods I learned about human anatomy, physiology, pathology, pharmacology, and various clinical sciences as to how to diagnose and treat various conditions. However, there was surprisingly very little education in the curriculum or the clinical training about death, dying, or end of life. The whole emphasis appeared to be the prevention of death and curing illnesses, but nothing about death itself. It was a matter to be dealt with by the community, church, or other religious organizations and family. Doctors do not talk about death even when they know it is impending and inevitable.

Venkit S. Iyer

I was the intern for the night duty when I witnessed the death of a person for the first time in my life. I can still remember the event. There was this elderly man in the ward who appeared to be having very labored breathing. I had no idea as to his medical history, or medical problems. There was no family at the bedside. The ward nurse appeared to be more cognizant of the situation than me. She told me this patient would be dying soon. I panicked and scolded her for inaction. I went to the bedside and examined him but had no clue as to what to do. I had just graduated from medical school, and it was my first night on call. I yelled at the nurse to do something and asked her to inject a respiratory stimulant immediately. It took nearly ten minutes before the medication could be brought from the pharmacy and injected. By that time the person had stopped breathing. I told the nurse that it was her fault that we could not give the injection any sooner and he could have been saved. At that time in the 1960s in India, we didn't know anything about CPR or intubation. The nurse had tears in her eyes from my panic and yelling because I was the doctor and she was a nurse. However, in reality, she had a more practical knowledge of having witnessed many deaths in the wards and it was a non-consequential incident. I was a novice who had never seen death previously.

Dying is a natural process. Many people consider that dying is a calamity, a bad thing that happens. It may be true if one dies prematurely from homicide or accident, but the death of an older person is often a relief and a matter of celebration. If someone dies of a terminal incurable condition such as cancer or degenerative disease, many are thankful for the end of suffering and agony. Imagine if no one died on this planet. We, humans, are already overcrowding this planet, taking over space from other animals. If no one died, we would be fighting for standing room. The nationalistic and isolationist policies would become more intense; there would be shortages of food and water, there would be more wars and environmental pollution.

Time goes only one way, always going forwards. We can go only forwards in time. No one can go backward in time to start over. So it is with the process of aging. It is a process that causes one to grow older and never younger and aging is bound to happen. The date of death is predestined for everyone, but that date and time is unknown. It is going to come, slowly or suddenly, knowingly or unknowingly, sooner or later, but it is certain to come. However, when the time comes everyone wants to be alive a little longer. Even with a chronic illness and anticipated terminal state, most families would say to the doctor, please do what you can, or try your best, or do anything possible, and the patient will say please don't give up on me. The medical science is full of doing fixes for the problem such as implanting a pacemaker for slow heartbeats or initiating dialysis for the kidney shut down or placing a ventilator for breathing problems and so forth. It is always fixing the short term and solving an immediate problem without addressing the person as a whole. So far, despite all the scientific knowledge and all the advances in medicine, it has not been possible to prevent death altogether. Death is inevitable. It is going to happen to every one of us, tomorrow or some other day in the future for sure.

Hinduism believes in the three phases of the life cycle, represented by three Gods, namely Brahma, Vishnu, and Siva. They stand for creation, preservation, and destruction. They also represent birth, life, and death. All three are important for the harmony of the universe. We can translate this to our body function such as eating, digesting, and eliminating as the three phases of nutrition that sustains life. If anyone of them is disrupted, the body suffers an illness. We may conclude that death is not bad after all.

Death is a great equalizer. No matter how rich or poor you were, no matter how good or how evil you were, no matter how famous or unknown you were it is a full stop for everyone. It ends there. You don't take anything with you, all the riches, all the luxuries, all the friends and families, your power, your glory everything ends. Those who are still alive may make something out of your estate, may construct a monument or a memorial, put up a statue or a painting or even write something about you, but it does not matter one bit as far as the dead person is concerned. It is a dark, oblivious, no return terminal event. No matter how carefully you plan it when the time comes, you go. You never know when the call comes: it may be by a stray bullet on the street, or a wrong-way driver or a heart attack, or lightning.

Tibetan Buddhists believe that every dying person goes through certain phases of dissolution, irrespective of how the person dies. First, the outer senses dissolve, making the person unaware of the five senses. Then four elements namely earth, water, fire, and air disappear one by one. When the earth dissolves the person cannot sit up when water dissolves all body fluids leak out, when fire disappears the body temperature plummets, and when air dissolves the person is gasping. Finally, the inner soul dissolves unseen by anyone returning to nature as one arrived from Nature. Ashes to ashes.

Chapter 18

HOW IS DEATH CONFIRMED

Years ago, it used to be fairly easy to call it, when people died in their homes. Grandma or grandpa stopped talking and breathing or did not wake up from sleep. They were living together in joint families. Sometimes they saw the elderly gasping for breath and poured some fluids into their open mouth. In India, it was customary to pour water from the Ganges they had saved in a sealed jar. The water is supposed to allow the person to go to heaven since it is sacred water. Often the individuals were unable to swallow the water or they aspirated it. After making sure that the person is completely unresponsive, they mourned around the body, bathed it, covered the body with fresh, new attire, and lit a lamp at the head. The funeral was cremation for the Hindus, and burials were for Muslims and Christians. There were no legalities, no death certificates, no registration in the county office, and no arguments about properties or inheritance. Everyone in the village knew everyone and everything and all residents participated in the funeral.

These days, things have become more complicated. We live in cities and we do not know our neighbors. Living in high-rise buildings, we do not know who is living next door or across the hallway. Things have become legal in every way. Often a reaction is out of fear or ignorance. First, we call 911 even when we know the person is expected to die with a terminal illness. Once the paramedics arrive, they take over the process. The family cannot even touch or mourn with the body. Even though we know the person is dead for sure, and even though the paramedics know the person is dead for sure, even though everyone was expecting the person to die from a long-standing illness, no one is willing to say the person is dead. Only doctors are allowed to say the person is dead.

They must then take the dead body in an ambulance to the nearest hospital, and have the doctor in the emergency room certify that the person is indeed dead. Then the body is kept in the mortuary until a death certificate is issued and formal funeral arrangements are made. This has to be done through a funeral home. The medical examiner has to give clearance. Then only formal mourning can take place and a formal funeral can take place. Following this, a legal protocol is observed to document the deceased person no longer exists and that the inheritances are allowed.

It is not that easy to confirm if a person is dead or not when the death is very recent. This is more so in the hospitals when the patient has been receiving multi-system life support. Several hours after death, it is much easier to say that there are no biological functions. In other words, no one can exactly and precisely state the exact second or minute when the patient actually died. Generally, in the hospitals, doctors wait around, conduct some tests and treatments, and finally set up a time arbitrarily when everyone has agreed it is futile to treat the person anymore. If the person dies on the regular floors or rooms, then they call "code", when a whole bunch of people run into the room, pump on the chest, give oxygen, and give all sorts of medications. Finally, they call it off after they have had an hour to reconfirm the person has been dead for certain. They document that time as "time of death" when they decided to call it off, and not the actual time when the person died. Truthfully speaking it is not important if someone is declared dead one or two hours after the actual event happens. Nothing much changes. It is more harmful to declare someone dead an hour or two earlier while the heart may still be beating. We are more interested in the exact time of birth as an important predictor of the baby's fortunes, but no one really cares as to the exact time of death, except for the medical examiner or coroner in cases of suspicious or violent deaths.

To define and confirm the death, doctors want to ascertain that there is no heart function, no lung function, and no brain function. To check the heart, they listen to the heart with a stethoscope, feel for the pulses over the carotid artery in the neck or the femoral pulses in the groin, and take a cardiogram or check the heart monitor on the wall. To check the lungs, they listen to the lungs with a stethoscope, check for breathing at the nose or mouth, and check the oxygen level with pulse oximetry. To check the brain function, they try to wake up the patient, cause severe pain by pressing against the eyeball, sternum, nail beds, or muscles. They touch the cornea and eyelids and check for muscle rigidity or flaccidity in the legs and arms.

Only when all of these three organ systems are fully non-functioning; only when they are certain; only when another individual has also independently agreed to these findings, only then do they issue the death certificate.

There are anecdotal stories that everyone has heard of when the dead body moves or stirs in the mortuary or the funeral home. There are also folk stories as to the exact events at the time of death. Some say they see a flame coming out of the mouth or chest at the moment when the soul leaves the body. Many have seen a dying person suddenly wake up, hold a person's hand or try to say something or roll their eyes, and then suddenly fall limp. In the movies, they add melodrama by showing the person suddenly roll the head to one side, or protrude the tongue out and lie still afterward. All of them claim to know the exact time of death, but with no scientific verification. According to Hindu mythology, Yama the God of death is supposed to take the soul from the body at a predestined time, arriving at the scene on top of a black buffalo. No one can see him, but some dogs and birds can see the arrival and they make ominous sounds just before the actual death.

These are just stories. In real life, as a physician who has practiced medicine for 50 years and who has done multiple lifesaving surgeries, I can vouch that it is difficult to state the very exact moment the person expires. We just approximate the time as close as reasonable.

Not everyone is afraid of dying. They are more afraid of how and when they die. We read about so many killings, accidents, and natural deaths. We read obituary as news. We always think that it is someone else, and deny that it is going to happen to us sooner or later. Buddhist philosophers believed that 'self' is an illusion and should not fear death. Hindus believe the real life is in the soul, which never dies, and it is using a human body for its purpose for a certain period. It is their opinion therefore that death never occurs. It is only an appearance or once again an illusion.

The science of organ transplantation and organ procurement has made it increasingly difficult and legalistic to define the actual time of death of tissues. There are horror stories of organs being harvested when the person is still alive. Moreover, it is possible to keep a body alive with artificial support of the lung, heart, and kidneys even when the brain is dead. The timing is important for organ procurement. If it is delayed too long the harvested organ will not be usable.

Sometimes, the hospital authorities or doctors decide to continue the artificial life support for political, legal, or financial reasons, knowing quite well that withdrawal of such support will cause immediate death. If a certain time interval is provided to prepare for the forthcoming bad news, to let the public and family know and give them a heads up, then it will be accepted with respect. A sudden and quick death is a shock and may at times end up in riots and calamity to the hospitals or doctors. Sometimes, it is because of a legal guardian or family member who has to agree to the withdrawal of life support, and the ethics committee of the hospital has to accept it. It is also known that certain unscrupulous doctors and hospitals have kept a dead body alive for an extra day or two for financial gains.

Criteria for establishing brain death were published in 2001. A qualified neurologist must do a complete neurological examination at a time when the core body temperature is normal, with no evidence of drug intoxication, poisoning, neuromuscular blocking agents, with no hypotension, normal electrolytes and acid-base balance, and no endocrine or metabolic disorders. The doctor should document deep coma, that there are no body reflexes, no corneal reflexes, no pain reactions, absence of brain stem reflexes, and apnea. Besides, certain confirmatory tests should be done. They are (1) Cerebral angiogram, which shows no intracranial filling, with patent extracranial vessels, (2) Electroencephalogram showing lack of reactivity to intense stimuli, (3) Transcranial Doppler Ultrasonography showing lack of diastolic flow, and (4) Cerebral Scintigraphy with technetium 99 showing the absence of blood flow. It is also wise to document a second opinion confirmation of brain death by another treating physician before the organ harvesting team is called in.

A recent experiment done at Yale University and published in Nature has provided some hope to restore brain function hours after clinical death. In this experiment, pigs that were killed in a food processing facility had their brains removed after four hours. These brains were then connected for six hours to a pump which delivered a special nutrient and chemical solution along with oxygen at the same rate as the normal heartbeat, and a had a filter resembling an artificial kidney, with temperature regulation. Afterward, the brains were checked for neuronal activity, focusing on the hippocampus area. They were shocked to see that the cells had preservation of the structure and were able to respond to tiny zaps of electrical signals. This is considered a revolutionary finding, which may redefine the timing of brain death. It may be a far off hope to reset brain function after stroke and head injuries, but it may change views on organ donation based strictly on brain death.

Chapter 19

HYPOTHERMIA

Hypothermia refers to low body temperature. It protects and prolongs life and also has the potential to save lives. However, excessive cold conditions can also cause death. The lowest recorded core temperature of a surviving adult was 60.8 degrees. Nazi doctors estimated that a 77degree core temperature would result in death. Women and children can survive cold temperatures better than men.

It has been demonstrated time and again that hypothermia or the cooling of the body preserves the brain function for longer periods than otherwise. Following CPR (Cardio Pulmonary Resuscitation), if the body is kept cool by using external measures such as ice packs or by internal measures such as infusing cold saline, there is a higher chance for them to recover. This should not be a surprising feature, since we commonly refrigerate food items, meat, and fish products for several days without any damage. People who died in high altitude mountains, covered with ice, are known to be preserved for extended periods. Mountain climbers on Everest have seen well-preserved dead bodies on the mountaintops. There have been many documented instances, where people who were considered to be dead have recovered completely if they were kept cool. It becomes premature to declare the time of death in these cases. Because of this feature, neurologists are cautioned to declare brain death only if the body temperature is normal or higher when they make such an evaluation.

Hypothermia is used as a way of keeping the body alive even after the heart has stopped beating, after the lungs have stopped breathing, and the brain appears to have gone into a state of unconsciousness. Medical technology in this aspect evolved many years ago. It buys time from the claws of death. The body slows down immediately, and the need for energy is reduced, and the metabolism breaks to slow pedal. The body keeps going on low fuel. According to a study, with a 1-degree drop in Celsius temperature, the body's need for metabolism goes down by 5 to 7%. When there is vasoconstriction, the blood vessels in the periphery of the body contracts, the blood is shifted to maintain core circulation- sending blood only to vital organs such as the heart, lungs, brain, and abdominal viscera, and it shuts off circulation to the rest of the body. Thus, it can prolong life beyond the normal.

Hibernation is a well-known phenomenon in the animal kingdom. During cold weather months, many animals dig themselves in and hibernate for long periods. Food is scarce and it is difficult to hunt. When the warm weather returns at the arrival of springtime they wake up. Polar bears cannot find food during the winter months. Ground squirrels are known to drop their heartbeats from 200 beats a minute to ten a minute during extreme cold weather periods and can hibernate for up to six months with no food or water.

This observation led scientists like Dr. Bigelow in 1950 to explore hypothermia for medical use. Dr. Norman Shumway and Dr. Richard Lower pioneered open heart surgery and heart transplantation in 1968, based on hypothermia as a mechanism to preserve body function. Now it is an accepted and standard modality used routinely in such operations. The body temperature is brought down to 28 degrees Celsius in a carefully monitored way.

When the body temperature is restored after a period of hypothermia, a serious adverse reaction can set in. It is similar to aftershocks following an earthquake or an ocean current pullback following a tsunami. The body swells up and fluid accumulates in the tissues. The brain becomes edematous or swollen and gets severely squeezed inside the tight non-yielding skull bone, which causes the brain death and death of the person. Many other parts of the body also get swelled up and there is a release of poisonous chemicals and enzymes, which lead to cell death. The whole body becomes mush. Hypothermia is good to prolong life, but rewarming can hasten death. Many of the deaths due to hypothermia occur during the rewarming period. Hence rewarming should be slow and carefully monitored.

This type of effect is commonly seen in peripheral vascular surgery practice. It is called reperfusion injury. For example, the circulation to a leg could be suddenly cut off from an embolus or a blood clot inside the artery. Gangrene will set in due to a lack of circulation if it is not corrected within six hours. The outcome is better if it is corrected early on. However, in practice, this is a difficult time goal, and a delay occurs due to any number of reasons. Let us say the corrective surgery took place and circulation got reestablished after a six-hour interval. The leg may survive, but it will swell up severely and go into a state that is called compartment syndrome. Doctors make long counter incisions all around the leg. It is called a four-compartment fasciotomy, to allow the muscles to bulge out. After several days, the tissues shrink, and the leg wounds either heal by themselves or can be closed separately. If such releasing cuts are not made, the tissues die inside and develop various nerve deficits and contractures. Sometimes they may develop further gangrene of the tissues despite the reestablished circulation, and still end up requiring an amputation. The poisonous toxins can get washed to the rest of the body and cause multi-organ damage such as kidney failure, or lung failure, or heart failure.

Similar effects are now recognized to take place inside the abdomen. Years ago, they were never recognized, and no one knew why a patient died despite corrective surgery. Now we know that Abdominal Compartment Syndrome (ABC) is a real phenomenon, where the entire abdominal cavity gets squeezed very tight inside due to the swelling of tissues. This affects internal blood flow further and the person goes into low blood pressure and low urine output. As a preventive measure, the doctors open up the abdomen and leave it open, cover it with a mesh or a cellophane type material. With time, the swelling recedes, and the person lives. Secondary closure of the abdominal wall is done afterward.

The problem with the brain is that the skull is a rigid bony cavity made to protect the brain. It is difficult to decompress the brain like the leg and abdomen. It is difficult to lay open the skull, even though parts of the skull bone are removed in a partial attempt for decompression. The better course of action is to keep the patient dry or dehydrated, while carefully monitoring the need for fluids. Sometimes they give diuretics or hypertonic solutions to dry out the brain tissues. Recovery from hypothermia must be slow, measured, and carefully monitored. It is better to keep the patient dehydrated rather than over hydrated.

Medical measures to rewarm the body includes placing the body inside warm blankets, body warmers that blow warm air under the sheets, giving warm intravenous fluids, and inserting a catheter in the urinary bladder to run warm irrigations. The ideal measure is to have a heart-lung bypass that infuses warmed blood back to the body. This may not be available in many regular hospitals. Another method is to place peritoneal dialysis catheters to infuse warm fluid into the abdominal cavity and then let them out.

In summary, hypothermia can protect life, but rewarming has to be carefully monitored. Death cannot and should not be confirmed when the body is in a state of hypothermia.

Chapter 20

WHAT CAUSES DEATH

The WHO (World Health Organization) study on May 24, 2018, showed 56.9 million people died a year worldwide. The top causes of death in the United State of America according to CDC as reported in March 2017 are:

- Heart disease
- Cancers
- Lung problems
- Accidents
- Stroke
- Alzheimer's disease
- Diabetes Mellitus
- Influenza and pneumonia
- Kidney Disease
- Suicides
- Preventable medical errors
- Drug addiction
- Homicides and gun violence

The causes of death can be differently classified as causes due to diseases, manmade disasters, natural disasters, and the natural process of aging.

Diseases: Ischemic heart disease and stroke were the biggest killers accounting for 15.2 million deaths. Other causes were a chronic obstructive pulmonary disease, lower respiratory infections, Alzheimer's disease, and dementia, cancers, diabetes mellitus, road accidents, diarrheal diseases, and tuberculosis.

Heart diseases: Heart diseases appear to take first place for causing death in all countries, all sexes, and all races. What exactly happens to the heart and why is it so vital to the body? It is the pump that keeps the circulation flowing. It is like the motor under the hood of the car. When it stops, the body tissues and cells do not get the oxygenated blood or nutrients that are needed to keep them alive.

The most common heart problem causing death appears to be blockage of the coronary arteries. We call this a heart attack. Like all other muscles and cells in the body, the heart itself has its muscle and tissues. The heart muscle gets its blood supply through the arteries called coronary arteries that arise from the very beginning of the aorta. When there is no blood to the heart muscle, it becomes weak and loses the muscle strength needed to push the blood to the rest of the body. Sometimes it is a massive and sudden blockage, causing sudden death. Sometimes it weakens only part of the heart muscle, making the person weak and incapacitated.

The most common reason for the blockage of the artery is a process called atherosclerosis. Plaques build up inside the lumen of the blood vessels. These plaques make the inside of the artery irregular and rough instead of remaining smooth. Slowly the plaques grow bigger becoming like coral reefs. Some of these plaques break off and float downstream and occlude the smaller branches. Sometimes they encourage clots to form and these clots occlude the lumen. Sometimes these plaques erupt like tiny volcanos and block the lumen.

Therefore, the question becomes what causes atherosclerosis. There are many risk factors we know of, but we still do not know the exact mechanisms. Genetic risk is certainly one factor. We have all heard of young people having heart attacks from time to time, as opposed to the usual pattern of older people getting heart attacks from blocked arteries. Diet is considered to be another factor. A high cholesterol diet, with animal fat, is supposed to be riskier.

Smoking, obesity, diabetes mellitus, inadequate exercise, stress, and uncontrolled high blood pressure and high blood cholesterol level are all risk factors. Despite all these precautions, still, the heart attack occurs due to unknown factors.

Many other problems can affect the heart. Cardiomyopathy is a state where the heart muscle is very flabby, and cannot contract with any force. The same occurs in congestive heart failure. It is like the motor running very slow and the car cannot pick up speed. The person is short of breath; fluid builds up in the tissues and lungs. Another situation is when the heart beats irregularly instead of regular normal beats. Sometimes the beats are so slow that the person has fainting spells, or sometimes it is a rapid beat that makes it inefficient and creates blood clots in the heart itself. Sometimes fluid builds up around the heart and chokes it, preventing it from proper heartbeats.

Lung disorders: The next set of problems leading to death are related to the lungs. When the lungs are not working properly, there is not enough oxygen mixing with blood and the tissues suffer. Lung problems can be sudden such as the collapse of a lung, or they can build up over a short period such as pneumonia or influenza or they can build up over many years such as asthma or emphysema. COPD (Chronic Obstructive Pulmonary Disease) is a term used to indicate a long-standing poor function of the lungs. Smoking, allergy, pollution, and heart conditions can certainly make things worse for the lungs. Cancer of the lung is a major killer. Even though we do not know of the reason for cancerous changes, it is proven beyond doubt that smoking will increase the chance of getting lung cancer.

Stroke: Stroke is paralysis with loss of function of one half of the body or weakness of one extremity along with slurring of speech or loss of memory or other neurological deficiencies. The most common cause of stroke is again atherosclerosis or hardening of the arteries. Plaques build up and block one of the internal arteries of the brain, cutting off circulation to one half of the brain or portion of it. Often the plaque buildup can be identified in the carotid artery in the neck, which can be treated by surgery or angioplasty. Once a stroke occurs, a series of further problems occur, such as balance problems, falls, ulcers in the back or buttocks, urinary infections, pneumonia, general weakness and malnutrition, and so forth. Something or another aggravates and expedites the end of life. The root cause is atherosclerotic plaques that build up. Smoking, obesity, diabetes, lack of exercise, bad diet, poor control of blood pressure, or other medical problems are the underlying risk factors.

Cancers: Cancers are the uncontrolled growth of cells in one part of the body, and they can spread to other parts also. The tumor applies pressure on normal organs and causes those tissues to suffer and they function poorly. Sometimes they cause bleeding or infection or blockage of tubular structures like intestines or bile ducts. Unless treated properly, most of them cause eventual death. We do not know why we get cancers. Many risk factors are identified, such as genetic abnormality, virus infection, diet, smoking, and certain drugs. If cancer is treated early on, there is a better chance for control or cure.

Diabetes mellitus: Diabetes Mellitus is a slow killer. The body is unable to metabolize sugar properly and leads to a variety of after-effects. Sometimes the blood sugar is very high and the body goes into a state of ketoacidosis, which can cause death. The blood vessels can narrow and plaque buildup occurs faster. Small-sized blood vessels occlude, resulting in gangrene and tissue necrosis. Wounds do not heal properly in diabetics. Nerves become damaged resulting in neuropathy or loss of sensations, resulting in wounds and ulcers. Kidneys stop working. The infections can spread deep inside the tissues without much visible change on the skin. Eyesight can be affected. The entire body is at a disadvantage and heart attacks and strokes lead to an earlier death than normal people.

Infections: Wide varieties of infections occur that can cause mortality. These include tuberculosis, HIV/AIDS, Ebola, malaria, cholera, viral infections, parasitic infestations, and bacterial infections.

80,000 people died in 2019 from flu attacks and related medical illness, and 900,000 people were hospitalized according to data published by the Center for Disease Control and Prevention. This was the highest level of flu-related deaths in four decades before this. Flu viruses mutate and produce a new strain every year. Flu vaccination is recommended for all even if it does not give complete immunity. It will reduce the severity of the infection and save lives.

A new pandemic caused by the Corona Virus (Covid-19) hit the world in 2020 and spread rapidly, making this infection a serious concern throughout the world. So far, it has infected over 50 million people worldwide in a short period of 9 months. It affected over 10 million people and killed over 230,000 people in the United States alone during this period as of the time of this writing. It is considered to be a mutant of a previous virus called SARS but has proven to be lethal for the elderly and medically disabled individuals. It spreads through air-born droplet contamination. When an infected person sneezes, coughs, laughs, or speaks aloud, the virus travels through the air and gets inhaled by others. Some infected people have very little symptoms whereas several others die very rapidly. In addition to the health care scare, the virus has caused a major dislocation to the economy due to the need for isolation, quarantine, and periods of lockdown and travel restrictions.

Chronic conditions: Dementia, Alzheimer's disease, bipolar disorder, and similar neurological problems are worse with increasing age, and lead to early death due to associated disabilities and accidents. The causes of these disorders are still unknown. Support from friends and families, and brain-stimulating activities, and certain medications are of some value.

Starvation: Starvation due to poverty, drought, and disasters and resulting malnutrition causes several people to perish. The sight of children suffering from malnutrition is heart rendering. Many lives are snubbed at a younger age just from lack of food and water in certain areas of the world, while the problem is obesity, waste, and abuse in other parts of the world.

Kidney Disease: Kidney failure can be sudden or acute related to shock, hypotension, severe dehydration, sudden blood loss, accidents and trauma or sepsis, infections, toxins, or reaction to medications. It can also slowly worsen or become chronic over several months or years due to a variety of illnesses such a diabetes mellitus, immune disorders, intrinsic renal disorders, or obstructive problems of the urinary tract. The sudden ones need intensive therapy with fluids or blood and at times diuretics or temporary dialysis. The long-standing kidney failures need close monitoring with medications, and may eventually end up with chronic hemodialysis. The ultimate treatment for them will be kidney transplantation. Kidney failure is a very common cause of death.

Preventable medical errors: Preventable medical errors are one reason for early death. Paradoxically, we go to the hospital to get well, but it is also a dangerous place to be. It is not intended that the doctors or hospitals make errors, but they do occur on a regular scale. Preventive health care in an outpatient setting is far superior to going to hospitals for treatment. Tests lead to more tests and procedures and they can snowball into a complication. Mistakes happen due to communication errors between different health care providers. Sometimes side effects of medications or antibiotics lead to more complications. All surgical procedures can lead to complications. Consumers are best advised to educate themselves, and by having family paying close attention to the care being rendered, while the primary care doctor oversees all orders every day while in the hospital.

Man-Made Disasters: Accidents, suicides, and homicides are man-made disasters. Nearly 50,000 people die each year in the United States of America from gun violence alone. 72,000 people died from a drug overdose and opioid addiction in the US in 2017. Another 50,000 people die from various accidents and traffic injuries each year in the USA. In a country such as India, it is estimated that 150,000 people die of road accidents every year due to poor road conditions, poor maintenance of vehicles, and driver fatigue and distraction, wherewith a certain amount of precaution these numbers can be reduced.

The easy availability of guns including military-style weapons leads to thoughtless and quick use of these weapons. It is well proven that in those countries where gun control is established, gun-related deaths are minimal. Stress reduction, family support, and mental health assistance can significantly reduce suicides, especially in the younger population age group. Avoiding driving under the influence of alcohol or drugs can reduce automobile accidents. Avoiding attention-diverting situations such as using cell phones, texting, eating, and sleeping while driving is also of value.

Natural Disasters: Large numbers of people are killed during natural disasters. These include hurricanes, tornadoes, earthquakes, wildfires, tsunamis, flooding, cyclones, and severe weather conditions. Hurricane Maria in 2017 caused over 3,000 people to die in Puerto Rico. The recent tsunami in Indonesia in September of 2018 caused over 2,500 people to die. Earthquakes have caused major disasters in Pakistan, Afghanistan, Ecuador, and Chile.

No one can identify the cause of natural disasters. Climate change and global warming are real events. They may also be due to changes in planetary alignments. Many believe that carbon pollution is affecting the ozone layer around the earth, causing these changes. If one believes in pre-historical mythology, there is confirmation that there was a deluge at some time in the past where most living creatures perished. There was an ice age where time was frozen. It is predicted that most people will die all across the globe from their misdeeds, and will result at the end of the world. Is it possible that there will be a major nuclear war attack between different countries, with most of mankind perishing from it? We will never know.

Natural Process of aging: Aging happens as a natural phenomenon. There is no single cellular event or change that happens to cause the cell to become aged or old. It is a combination of multiple small little changes that accumulate over a while. We can postulate that the DNA has to continue to make the same sequence of molecules inside the chromosome for it to continue to function. When one of the molecules fails to register in the sequence that particular chromosome tends to become unhealthy. The enzyme telomerase is considered to be necessary to create this repetitive molecular sequencing. Why does the telomerase enzyme go down and what can be done to keep it flowing? Other than theories and suggestions, we still do not know the reasons for aging.

We have to go into the microscopic structure of the cell to see when and how it dies. Cell death is called apoptosis. It is considered as a physiologic phenomenon, where there is a disruption of cell membrane and disruption of a chromosome. Inside of the chromosome DNA replication occurs which is controlled by telomeres. After a few replication cycles, the ends of DNA strands lose their ability to replicate which leads to cell death. Telomerase activity is high in the embryonic cells and stem cells. They are also high inside the cancer cells, which explain the growth of the cancer tumor.

Therefore, we end up saying that a certain person died of old age. No special reason like a heart attack or stroke. We accept that the person has been slowly withering away little by little. The hearing lowers, eyesight weakens, joints creak, back pain becomes frequent, people may not urinate properly, or sleep properly, the appetite may be reduced, weight may be lost, so on and so forth. The person may need help with day-to-day functions. Initially, it may be difficult to travel, then driving and shopping, and later cooking and getting dressed. Eventually, the person requires help for personal needs such as using the toilet and bathing. Why does the aging occur, why does the body stop functioning even when there is no one single reason to pinpoint? We still do not know the exact process of aging of the cells of the body. We know it happens and that eventually death occurs no matter how much medical science has advanced or holds promises for the future.

Chapter 21

MASS CASUALTIES

When large numbers of people die from one event, one disaster, one war, or by one murderer, it leaves a big impact on the society, as compared to a single individual dying one at a time from old age or illness. We not only want to sympathize with the victims, but we also want to express our anger against the person who caused it. We wonder how we could have prevented it and what we can do to prevent such incidents in the future. However, the number of people dying one at a time far exceeds the number of people dying in mass casualties. A single incident causing the death of 10 or 20 people at a time causes a shock wave, but over 72,000 people dying from opioid overdose each year is unrecognized.

Mass casualties can be due to natural disasters, man-made disasters, or accidents. Natural disasters are items such as hurricanes, typhoons, tsunamis, earthquakes, tornadoes, volcanoes, floods, mudslides, and wildfires. Premeditated human disasters include wars, famines, riots, racial violence, mass shootings, terrorism, and ethnic cleansing. Then there are accidents such as plane crashes, boats capsize, overcrowding and stampedes, bus accidents, and train accidents to mention a few.

Natural disasters: Natural disasters bring in the power of Mother Nature to an amazing level that makes humans humble. The earth is still a molten liquid in its core and the continents are still shifting. Many more people used to die from natural disasters in the past since there were no forewarnings and people were unprepared. That has improved in modern times, with much-improved weather forecasting and public warnings. Still, in 2017, hurricane Maria caused the death of over 3,000 people in Puerto Rico. Hurricane Katrina in 2005 caused 1,833 deaths in New Orleans.

Volcanic eruptions have buried whole cities in the past. Pompeii in Italy was buried under several feet of ashes and lava. Volcanic mudflow or landslide is called a lahar. In 1985, in Armero such a tragedy caused the death of 23,000 people.

Tsunamis occur when there is an underwater earthquake, which displaces a large volume of water, causing huge tidal waves. In 2004, the Indian Ocean tsunami started near Sumatra, Indonesia, with damage to 14 countries and an estimated death toll of 280,000 people. The Indonesian islands are prone to repeated incidences of earthquakes and tsunamis. The last one that happened in late September of 2018 resulted in nearly 2,000 deaths.

Wildfires cause major damages to people, property, and land. Wildfires in California have been devastating. The fires in Paradise, California in November 2018 caused 79 people to die and 1,000 people missing over an area size of the city of Chicago in just two weeks.

A major cyclone by the name of Idai caused havoc in Mozambique in March of 2019. It was a sudden tropical cyclone that devastated towns and killed nearly 200 people overnight. It spotlighted how rapid urbanization and climate change can turn deadly. 90% of a city by name of Beira was destroyed with winds over 100 miles per hour along with rains and floods.

There is room to discuss whether natural disasters have something to do with climate change or not. No doubt that there are global warming and the melting of the glaciers. There is adequate and obvious proof for the same. We are also experiencing extreme temperature changes recently with severe cold spells in the northern USA, causing the death of over 10 people in January 2019, and at the same time temperature over 120 degrees in Australia and India. There have been too many incidents of severe rainfall and draught at the same time during the past year. It may be related to human pollution of the planet or it may be due to planetarium alignment changes.

The United Nations report submitted through a joint effort by a group of 90 scientists from 40 countries predicted recently that there could be a culmination of the greenhouse effect that will cause severe weather changes resulting in major disruptions in the world by 2040. Proof exists that extreme drought in certain parts of the world like South Africa and Sudan and severe floods and rains in other parts of the world as well as the melting of polar ice provides real evidence of this.

Man-Made Disasters: Man-made disasters occur when there are willful mass murders. These occur as a result of war, racial violence, ethnic disputes, partitions of countries, terrorism, and gun violence. Wars and killings of humans have been going on from prehistoric times. It is only the humans who kill each other for fun, control, power, religion, and race. No other creatures of the animal kingdom do killings for these reasons. They kill for food and sex, which are biological needs. Over a million people died following the partition of India and Pakistan. The Hindu Muslim conflict was inflated based on the desire for political and geographic control by the newborn nations. The fight for Kashmir continues after three wars.

During 1965-66, 400,000 to 3 million people were massacred in Indonesia to eliminate communists. In 1948-51 during the Korean War over 200,000 were killed. In 1645-46 the Sichuan massacre occurred, killing 1 to 3 million Sichuan's people by the army of Zhang Xianzhong in China. In 1182, 60,000 to 80,000 Latins were massacred by mobs in Constantinople.

During the civil war in Sri Lanka, between1970 to 1990 over a million people died, when there were conflicts between the Buddhist (Sinhalese) groups and Tamil groups (known as LTTE or Tamil Tigers).

Most people think that Adolf Hitler who executed the Jews was the biggest murderer. Hitler killed 6 million Jews along with 250,000 gypsies and another 250,000 homosexuals, and 70,000 mentally retarded or disabled people as unworthy of living. Others think it was Joseph Stalin, but it was Mao Zedong who caused the death of nearly 45 million people in China between 1958- 1962 during his dictatorship, in the name of the Great Leap Forward policy. He has been the biggest murderer in world history. However, this does not get recognition since it was reported to be due to famines, forced labor, and the death of peasants in remote villages.

In 1992 Bosnia- Herzegovina declared independence. Afterward, there was an effort to expel Bosnian Muslims. Over 8,000 people were killed in the town of Srebrenica in 1995. In 1994 ethnic cleansing took place in Rwanda when the majority Hutus massacred thousands of minority Tutsis. In 2003, Sudan split and hundreds of thousands perished in the Darfur area. During the terrorist attack of the 9/11 bombing of the World Trade Center in New York, the impact left a gaping, burning hole near the 80th floor of the 110-story skyscraper, instantly killing hundreds of people and trapping hundreds more on higher floors. Nearly 3,000 Americans died that day during the airborne terrorist attacks that hit the twin World Trade Center Towers, the Pentagon, and the thwarted attack of Flight 93 causing President George Bush to declare war against terrorism, with the invasion of Iraq and Afghanistan. This has taken an extreme toll since both directly or indirectly as ISIS was formed in the aftermath. The fights continue all over the Middle East and over a million have perished so far in the last 16 years and millions more were made homeless and destitute.

Korea has been receiving a fair amount of attention recently. When one looks back, the Korean War that lasted three years from June 1950 to July 1953, resulted in the death of over 1.2 million soldiers and nearly 2 million civilians, which was all a power grab between the US, Russia, and China following the Second World War.

Killings are expected to be a part of the life cycle as decided by nature when we look at killings from a different angle. Animals specifically kill the weaker ones for food and sexual partners. They kill when they are threatened or fear of their own life as a defense. Humans kill plenty of animals after feeding them and nursing them. They raise fish farms, chicken farms, and cattle farms, to kill them mercilessly, for food and other products such as leather and ivory for economic gains. Humans also kill animals for pure fun and sport unlike other animals, but they also killed other humans for slaves, sex, control, and power. Killings are a way of life for humans.

Famines have been created by willful maneuvers of dictators and politicians or wars. Thousands of people perish during the famines due to hunger and malnutrition. In 1943, Winston Churchill denied food supplies to villagers in Bengal on the pretext of the needs of the military troops. It is reported that at least one million people died of starvation in India that one year alone. Famines have occurred in Sudan, Myanmar, and several other African countries caused by dictators.

In Mexico, nearly 40,000 people go "missing" every year due to violence, kidnappings, and murders. Over 1,500 mass graves have been identified, and about 250,000 people are feared dead in just the last 10-year period. Families are afraid to report the missing, for fear of more repercussions. This is referred to as a crisis of culture in Mexico.

Mass graves and memorials can be seen all over the world. Ultimately it is the extreme desire for power, control, and money that motivates these crimes.

Environmental pollution: Large numbers of people die every year due to environmental pollution. A WHO study released in October 2018 shows that 7 million are dying every year from air pollution alone. This is created by carbon emissions and other factory outlet emissions. The greenhouse effect causing damage to the ozone layer is real. Air pollution is very severe in big cities such as New Delhi, Beijing, and many of the under-developed world. In addition, pollution of the waterways and rivers added with the lack of drinking water causes communicable diseases such as cholera, dysentery, and other parasitic infestations. Pollution of the surroundings with lack of garbage disposal, lack of sanitary facilities, and toilet facilities add to the disasters. If only we can focus on reducing pollution all around us including air, water, and food, and be aware of clean living and sanitary conditions we can save millions of lives from premature deaths.

Pandemics: From time to time the world has seen the rapid spread of communicable diseases killing hundreds of thousands of people in a short time. These infections that spread globally are called pandemics. Bubonic plague, anthrax, smallpox, and viral infections have caused millions to perish. Spanish flu in 1918, after the first world war killed 50-100 million people worldwide. It was a new strain of a virus that came from birds and medical science was underdeveloped at that time. The new pandemic that is causing great havoc today is the coronavirus/Covid-19 infection, which started in the Wuhan district in China less than a year ago. In this short time, it has already killed over 1 million people worldwide and has caused massive socio-economic damage everywhere.

Chapter 22

NEAR DEATH EXPERIENCES (NDE)

In his book "Last Breath: Cautionary Tales from the Limits of Human Endurance", Peter Stark describes several situations and examples where people were considered dead when they were pushed to the edge and were then brought back following the extremes of human endurance. He describes hypothermia due to freezing in the snow, drowning, mountain sickness, avalanche, scurvy, heatstroke, falling from heights, animal predators, the bends, cerebral malaria, and dehydration, all in real-life experiences, where they met death and were miraculously rescued.

It is well known that some people on certain occasions have experienced death and then returned to normal life. They give a wide range of exhilarating experiences. It is like going into a deathbed and getting life back. People have literally died under anesthesia during a complicated surgery, or major trauma, where all doctors and nurses had given up hope, but they hang on by a thread and come back to life. People have had cardiac arrests when the heart had stopped totally and came back. During heart surgery and heart transplantation, the body is kept alive with an external pumping mechanism. People who had deep hypothermia can be in hibernation for an extended period. It is estimated from polls that nearly 13 million Americans have experienced a Near Death Experience (NDE) in their life.

Such an occurrence is described in the Hindu mythology story of Savithri and Satyvan. She married him being in love, even though she knew that his life would be short. She performed serious prayers and pious meditations. Because of her virtuosity, and on the day of her husband's death, she was able to see the God of Death called Yama arriving on a black buffalo. She was able to see him and talk to him because of her pious and sacred nature. She pleaded with him to release her husband's life, but Yama told her that the day and time of death are always predetermined and there was no way to change that eventuality so she followed him to the outer world. Yama tried his best to shirk her off his trail telling her she is not allowed in there since her time has not arrived. However, because of her perseverance and persistent pleadings, Yama was forced to let go of her husband Satyavan and thus she was able to bring him back to life and they lived for many years together. A modern-day explanation for this story could be that Satyavan had a near-death experience and Savithri was able to bring him back with excellent care.

In another Hindu mythology story, a very honest and righteous king by the name of Harischandra was tested to the extreme by the demigods, who felt he was getting more praise and recognition than themselves. He was made to relinquish all his possessions and kingdom to keep his words and uphold honesty. Eventually, a snake bit his son and he died soon. The king was forced to cremate his son's body. As he was about to lite the funeral pyre, the supreme God appeared in front of him, and apologized on behalf of the demigods, and returned his kingdom and wealth, and gave back his son's life. The son woke up from the funeral pyre and they lived happily ever after. It is quite possible that the son had a near-death experience from the snakebite, and that he recovered from it.

Those who have experienced near-death describe a softly illuminated flame-like figure making them feel peaceful and comfortable. They did not experience pain during this phase. After their recovery, they did not recall bad experiences or painful matters. They felt rejuvenated and refreshed. They found themselves to be more mellow, stress-free, and soft. Some say that they could hear things others were saying, while they were still in a deep state of unconsciousness. They could sometimes feel that people were moving around them.

Their experiences confirm that death does not happen in an instant. It appears to be a slow process, which can be stopped at times, or reversed. It is difficult to define when death has taken place. Even after the doctors have declared that there is no spontaneous heart function, lung function or brain function there appears to be a period that exists before the irreversible mortality sets in. This twilight phase can be prolonged by cooling the body or inducing a coma, where the person can be brought back from the door of death.

The fact is that certain body parts can suffer from the poor blood supply and progressively deteriorate where that part can die. Also, the blood supply can be restored to that body part by surgery, or stents, or sometimes medications. This is called ischemia-reperfusion. It is the bringing back of blood to the area that was deprived of it. There are a series of severe changes that occur to that body part in this process. They swell up, for example, there can be patches of dead tissue among surviving tissues. Several days are required for them to settle down. Now, take the same example to the whole body, when the heart completely stops, and there is a loss of blood supply to the brain and other organs. When the heartbeat is reestablished following CPR or other measures, circulation is reset, but the body had nearly died already, and it is trying to come back to life. The body has to go through an injury path to recover and regenerate, which can take many days. We can call this an example of a near-death experience.

Then there have been many stories and news events when people who were considered to be dead or passed have been saved. On September 24, 2018, CNN carried the story of a 74-year-old male who was saved from a burned-out apartment building in Washington DC. He was trapped inside the apartment for over 5 days and was considered dead. The doors were jammed and would not open due to the swollen beams from the heat. The firemen broke open the door with crowbars, to inspect the inside, and found the man barely alive.

There was a long drama of several boys and their coach belonging to a boy-scout camping tour in Thailand in July of 2018, publicized on live television all over the world. They were trapped inside a cave for many days without water or food. The cave was flooded and there was no escape. After many days of search, the rescue crew found them, but the steps to save them were very difficult. Lifeguards and navy seals from different countries participated in a drill that lasted for several more days. Eventually, the heroic measures paid off, and all the boys and the coach were saved.

Experiences in the war fields, adventure trips, and mining expeditions have similar stories to tell. They had all experienced near death and saw God at times. Once saved, they became sober and spiritual.

In another movie called "Hereafter", very visual scenes are shown where people die during a tsunami in Thailand. With the actual dying process of a woman, what she goes through, what she experiences, how her body washes ashore, how she is given CPR, and considered to be dead, and how she breaths again and comes back to life are shown graphically. They experience peace and see a transformative and positive experience in life afterward. They become more altruistic, less materialistic, more detached, and less afraid.

In 1975, Raymond Moody published the book "Life after Life" in which he described experiences of nearly 150 people who had near-death experiences. His definition of NDE was a clinical situation that would have led to death without immediate medical intervention. They start out hearing a loud noise and moving through a dark tunnel. Afterward, they describe a feeling of peace, happiness, and being pain-free. Some felt they were floating up, looking down on their own body. Some experienced a panoramic view of their lives and the milestones in their lives, including memorable events. Some saw their dead family members welcoming them. Some recall a bright light and going through a tunnel. Some saw a beautiful domain with a luminous figure showering absolute love and compassion. They were reluctant to return to life, leaving behind an incredibly beautiful scene. All of them had changed drastically afterward, in their attitude, behavior, belief, and temperament.

In his book "Proof of Heaven", Dr. Eben Alexander, a Harvard trained neurosurgeon describes his own near-death experience, after contracting E-coli meningitis. He says he saw a bright light with great peace and serenity and met his sister whom he had never met previously, but who had already died."

In these near-death experiences, one is led to believe that the soul and body are separate entities. As described in almost every ancient scripture, the soul separates and reenters the body when the near-death experience is over, making the Deadman live.

Could it be possible that certain chemicals are released in the neural cells in the brain at the time of death to numb the effects of the upcoming calamity in the form of death? We know that such chemicals do exist to make us feel good in times of severe strain to the body. For example, the chemical called endorphins is released during concentrated physical activity such as long-distance running or competitive tennis games. They do not feel any pain and move spontaneously with minimal effort. When asked how they did it the usual answer is that they did not know. They were "in the zone" where things happened.

Other chemicals are known to influence the brain from feeling good to levels of hallucinations. Serotonin, dopamine, alcohol, ketamine, cocaine, phencyclidine (LSD), amphetamines, are all drugs or chemicals that have varying effects. When there is poor circulation and there is anoxia in the brain cells, some of these chemicals could be released to make the person feel good in spite of severe adversity the body is facing. It may be the body's mechanism to blunt the effects of impending disaster. Another psychedelic drug is DMT (Dimethyltryptamine). A small amount of it is naturally produced in the brain, but under intense bodily stress, a larger amount is released through the pineal gland, inducing the near-death experience and related comfort zone.

Miracles do happen from time to time and these episodes make one think and realize how little we know by way of science. There are many stories of advanced cancer that have been felt to be incurable and terminal, with miraculous remissions and near-complete recovery. Something in the body changes suddenly, it may be the immune system or it may be cellular regeneration. When these events occur, we pray and place our faith in God or superpowers.

Near-Death Experience (NDE) is separate from a Real Death Experience. The NDEs give us a collective subconscious memory of what happened to them in a state of critical illness. No one has given us a real death experience, since the person is dead and cannot talk. How many facts and truths are there in the NDEs is open for discussion. Some of it may be real; some of it may be hallucinations, some of it may be fragmented memory of events and talks, some of it may be pure imagination. Despite various claims, one can say that near-death experiences do not categorically equate with afterlife events or information.

Suspended animation is a term used where someone is lingering without being aware of oneself, almost dying but still alive and can be revived. It is a hypometabolic state created to have a temporary cessation of all body functions including the brain. It is sometimes referred to as hibernation. It can be induced with the use of hypothermia, cryotherapy, or chemicals.

Chapter 23

HOW SHOULD WE DIE

This is the true story of a doctor I knew, who lived and worked in my neighborhood. He was a pulmonary specialist and intensive care specialist, who would treat critically ill patients. He was in his late 50's and worked very hard day and night with no time to take care of himself. He was losing weight and was having abdominal pain and when it became unbearable, he saw a gastroenterologist. Tests showed he had advanced cancer of the stomach, which had spread, to the liver and the rest of the abdomen. It was incurable by all accounts with a high chance of death within a few weeks. They decided surgery was unnecessary and meaningless. Therefore, they decided on chemotherapy, which has no value and is toxic. In the next few weeks, he became debilitated and developed severe abdominal pain. They took him to the hospital emergency room, where an X-ray showed the cancer had made a hole in the stomach. Once the patient is in the emergency room, all prior opinions and thoughts are disregarded as the patient is unable to make any comprehension, and the family is lost. They let the emergency room and hospital doctors do what they felt was best. This now became a legal formality and the on-call surgeon decided to operate on the patient with the diagnosis of a ruptured stomach. During surgery, he did a complex resection of the stomach and placed multiple bags and tubes. After surgery, the patient did very poorly and had various complications, and went into multiple organ failures. The doctor was admitted to the intensive care unit of the same hospital where he used to work, with all sorts of drips and tubes, bloated like a frog, unable to talk, communicate or be aware of his surroundings. Every different specialist was called in for numerous tests, and no one wanted to give up, doing the maximum for their fellow colleague, with no one wanting to take any full responsibility either. The family was totally lost. After three weeks of a vegetative state, at the consensus suggestion, they decided to stop life support and he finally expired the following day.

This is not an uncommon scenario. No matter how busy you are, how good you are, and how important you are, you must take of yourself. You can help others only if you are in good health yourself. This person had decided against surgery, but then why take toxic chemotherapy when you know it has no value and it can only cause more harm. Then he was taken for surgery at the worse time, in his worse medical condition, with worse outcomes. Once you are in the hospital, no one uses common sense since everyone wants to work within their specialties, and meet the legalities and formalities, so instead of dying in peace with dignity at his home with his family at his bedside, he dies in the hospital after many more weeks of suffering from tubes all over the body, unable to talk or communicate during the last days of his life. We do not know if there was a Living Will or not, but there is enough evidence to say that initially, he had decided against unnecessary treatments. If the family and patient do not make firm decisions, the emergency room and hospitals will keep working, since no one wants to make a mistake and no one wants to be blamed for negligence or inadequate care.

Death is inevitable and everyone born to this world is going to die one day or another. However, our perception of how we die and what is a good death has changed over time. If we consider that humans are part of the biological world, where all living creatures that are born will die, then the same rule should apply to humans as well. There is no rule set by nature that all humans must die in a hospital or nursing home. They can die in their homes as they did decades ago.

There is also no rule set by nature that death should be slow and prolonged over a course of several days or weeks as we see today. If there is adequate time given to family and friends to absorb the news of impending death, they had adequate time to express sympathy, then we consider that as a good death, a natural death, and an expected one.

If the death is sudden and unexpected, then it is considered unnatural.

There was a time when everyone wanted to die quickly and suddenly so that they can depart this world with minimal suffering and leave without being a burden to the family or society. A quick death was considered as a good death then. Women wanted to die before their husbands so that they would not be branded as widows in the society. However, this attitude has changed, to the extent that sudden deaths are investigated to make sure there was no foul play. When the police arrive, often the spouse is the first suspect.

There was a time when family members cared for elderly individuals in their homes. There was good social interaction between residents in the same village and everyone cared for each other, everyone knew about each other. Elderly individuals were expected to die in their beds, with minimal suffering giving little troubles to their caregivers. Friends and extended family members made an effort to visit the elderly and sick just for the sake of visiting them. There was no need for a death certificate, will, or medical investigation. Everyone accepted that it was time for the person to go and conducted a funeral and the rest of the family moved on.

During my practice, I have seen numerous patients whom we considered as "vegetating", and felt sorry for them. These were patients who were bedridden and were unable to take care of themselves in any manner. Some of them had contractures of hip and knee and were lying like a pretzel. When the nurses try to turn them from one side to the other, the whole body has to be turned as a stiff object, bent at the knee and hip. They had multiple deep decubitus ulcers over the back in the coccygeal area and the trochanteric areas. They often make incomprehensible sounds at times or were in a subconscious state. However, they would swallow pureed food if fed with a spoon and would lie in their stools or urine until one of the nursing aids came over to clean them. They were sent to nursing homes and then back to the hospital for issues such as fever, urinary tract infections, or pneumonia. Without family involvement in their daily care, no visitors, no flowers at the bedside, the chart would indicate that the next of kin is residing out of state, and/or has given the power of attorney to a local guardian. The legal guardian would usually say, "Do what is medically right" even though there is a Living Will. The doctors would continue to treat since there is Medicare coverage. Eventually one day the patient dies as unknown individuals, alone, with the next of kin showing up mainly for the legal formalities and to collect the estate. This type of death we accept as normal or expected for many individuals in our society.

Then there are many individuals whom I have seen dying in the Intensive care unit, after several days and weeks of acute care. It was appropriate to give full throttle medical care at the onset of their illness. However, after a period of two or three weeks, everyone seems to lose sight of the big picture and continues to focus on the last few hours or the last day in making the next medical decisions. Correction of blood gases and electrolytes are made; then intravenous nutrition and an adjustment of ventilator settings and cardiac monitoring. However, no one seems to know what and why some things are being done. The electronic medical records repeat information already known and ends with "continue present treatment". Physicians and nurses as well as technicians are all working in shifts, and want to pass the buck over to the next person. Family is often lost in the conundrum of activity and is encouraged to say, "Yes" to all suggestions. They are afraid that they may offend someone otherwise, and they do not want to interfere with physician recommendations. The only person who can see the big picture is the primary care physician or the insurance company who is covering the expenses until eventual pressure comes down from hospital administration when there is no more money to be made. By this time the patient has gone into multiple organ failure, is bloated up, and has needles and tubes in every imaginable orifice. Then permission is asked from the family or legal guardian to "pull the plug" or stop life support. This type of death is also what we consider as normal or expected in modern times.

Now and then the moralists, legalists, and right-to-life advocates get involved in the private life of the person and with the family to decide what is good for the society in their view. We have heard the stories of Karen Ann Quinlan and Terry Schiavo cases when the Government and right to live advocates interfered with family decisions regarding allowing the person to die in dignity when there was no hope of survival or no quality of life left.

KAREN ANN QUINLAN CASE:

In 1975, a 21year old young lady, Karen Ann Quinlan went into a coma after consuming certain drugs and alcohol at a party. She was considered brain dead and was supported with a breathing machine. After one and a half months, the family was told by the neurologist that she was in a permanent vegetative state and there was no hope of returning to normal function. Her lower brain or brain stem was working to keep her alive, but the upper brain was nonfunctional. She could make some movements and make some noise, but she had to be supported with respirator and tube feedings. After several more months of such treatment, and many discussions and evaluations, consultations with clergy and attorneys, the family wanted the ventilator to be disconnected. However, the hospital and the doctors refused, stating that it would be equal to intentional killing.

The parents filed a lawsuit in Morristown, New Jersey, requesting the father be appointed as legal guardian and permission be given to withdraw life support. Such a case was unprecedented in the US and received wide media publicity. This was complicated by various media publicity showing a school photo of a beautiful looking young lady on one side, claims of her being alive on the other side, hitherto unknown documentation of Living Will, right to life groups, and right to die groups hashing their arguments. The court had appointed a temporary guardian in the meantime. He and the hospital argued that their job was to do everything possible to keep her alive as dictated by moral values and that the parent's request was equal to mercy killing.

Judge Muir made the verdict on November 10, 1975, denying permission to withdraw life support and the respirator as well as denying the request of the father to be legal guardian, stating that it would not be in the best interests of the victim. He stated that the parent couldn't request the death of an incompetent child. Karen's intentions were not clearly documented and it would be best to leave the decisions of care under the hands of treating doctors.

The case was appealed and went to New Jersey Supreme Court in January of 1976. On March 31 of 1976, the Supreme Court reversed the verdict of the lower court. It ruled on behalf of the family, appointing the father as the legal guardian and allowing legal immunity to the hospital from disconnecting the respirator if they decided to do so.

However, the hospital still refused to disconnect the respirator but did start weaning her off the breathing machine by turning it off for longer and longer seconds. Meanwhile, the family researched and had her transferred to a nursing home with advanced care. On June 9, 1976, she was transferred to Morris View Nursing Home. Here finally, the respirator was disconnected, except she started breathing on her own defying the expectations that she will die soon. She was kept alive by tube feedings and intravenous fluids and antibiotics. Her family wanted to continue these measures. After ten years of being in a vegetative state, she finally expired from pneumonia on June 13, 1986.

The Quinlan case was a turning point in the history of American medicine. There was no legal precedence of advance directives, Living Will, or right to die. Great awareness was brought in to hospitals, physicians, and people across the country. As a result, all the states in the US have introduced bills allowing advanced directives and a durable power of attorney. Currently, all the hospitals in every state in the USA now respect these directives. The right to refuse treatment, the right to die, and the right of the legal guardians to make decisions are accepted without question. Everyone recognizes the need to avoid unnecessary costs and suffering in the last days of life. Ethics committees are established in all hospitals across the country to discuss difficult situations and to give guidance to physicians and families. Almost everyone agrees to the undesirability of having a legal fight and court challenges regarding the end of life care.

The American Medical Association changed its position in 1986, stating that it is ethically permissible for physicians to stop respirator and feeding tube on someone in a permanent vegetative state (PVS) if the family or legal guardian wanted it so. In 1980, the Catholic Church, the staunchest of all right to life advocates, accepted that patients have the right to refuse medical treatment provided death is imminent and treatment is futile, through a declaration by Pope John Paul II.

TERRY SCHIAVO CASE:

Terry Schiavo was only 26 years old when she suffered cardiac arrest in 1990. There was no foul play and it was noted that she was bulimic and was dehydrating herself. When she was taken to the hospital after 911 was called, she was found to have severe hypokalemia (low potassium), which may have triggered her cardiac arrest. She had irreversible anoxic brain damage by then and was declared to be in a persistent vegetative state (PVS) after two months of intensive care.

In 2003 national attention reached a peak with this case with massive media attention due to a fight between right to life and right to die groups, multiple lawsuits, and political drama. She was in a vegetative state for over ten years, when her husband wanted to respect her verbal wishes by stopping her tube feedings. However, her parents wanted the feeding continued and went to court. The problem was that Terry Schiavo had not signed a written Living Will or durable power of attorney. By the common law convention, the care and legal proxy was the husband who was indeed providing good care.

This was complicated by the fact that she had certain involuntary eye movements, and a photograph taken in certain angles made it appear as if she was looking at you. Her upper brain had completely stopped working but some areas of the brain stem were still alive. These involuntary motions were interpreted as a living person and the effort to remove the feeding tube was interpreted as euthanasia.

In 1998, Michael Schiavo petitioned the sixth circuit court to have the tube feedings stopped. The parents opposed this. In April 2001 the feeding tube was removed but then it was reinserted 7 days later by an appeals court. It was again removed in 2003. Immediately, the Florida legislature passed "Terri's Law" signed by Governor Jeb Bush, and the tube was reinserted. In 2004 Judge Baird declared that Terri's Law was unconstitutional and the Florida Supreme court concurred. In 2005 Judge ordered the tube removed.

The US Congress passed a special expedited one-day bill allowing her parents to keep her alive, by transferring the case to the Federal court system from the Florida courts. President George Bush flew overnight from Texas to Washington DC just to sign the bill. Senators expressed much emotion, without examining the patient or looking over details. The dispute was heard in Federal courts and finally reached the US. Supreme court, which ruled in favor of the husband.

The feeding tube was removed eventually on March 18, 2005, and she died peacefully on March 31st, 2005. The parents would not let it go and wanted an autopsy which once again confirmed no hope for life and no foul play. She had severe anoxic brain damage with no function at all. Their fight continued to the funeral and book publications and media contests afterward.

NANCY CRUZAN CASE:

On the night of January 11, 1983, Nancy Beth Cruzan, a 25-year-old Missouri woman lost control of her car and landed face down in a water-filled ditch. By the time paramedics arrived, she had already developed anoxic brain damage. Since her brain stem was still working, she was able to breathe on her own, but was in a permanent vegetative state. She had to be kept alive with tube feedings.

After four years of treatment due to lack of improvement, Cruzan's parents wanted to stop the tube feedings, but the physicians and hospital refused since there was no written Living Will by Cruzan. The lower court judge granted this permission to the parents based on verbal testimony by her friends who had conversations with her about her desire against prolonging life in situations like this.

However, the State of Missouri appealed the decision and in November of 1988, the Supreme Court of Missouri reversed the lower court decision, granting the State's unqualified interest in preserving life, and wanted clearer evidence of Nancy Cruzan's wishes.

The Cruzan's appealed the case to the US. Supreme court, which heard it on December 6, 1989, and eventually, made the final ruling on June 25, 1990, which affirmed the right of a competent adult to refuse treatment of incompetent wards but agreed with the Missouri Supreme Court to show clearer evidence of Nancy's wishes. Hence the feeding tube could not be removed.

The Cruzan's returned to Missouri for a new trial in November 1990. This time more friends of Nancy's came forward and testified that Nancy had made very clear statements against being kept alive under a vegetative and unconscious condition. The State of Missouri withdrew its opposition at this point. Nancy's feeding tube was removed on December 14, 1990, and she died on December 26, 1990, almost 8 years after the initial accident.

As a result of the wide publicity from the Cruzan case and Quinlan case, greater awareness and interest occurred for having Living Wills and advance directives all across the country. Congress passed the Patient Self Determination Act, which requires all health care institutions to inform patients of their right to fill out advance directives and explain the policies. The right to refuse not only medical treatment but also nutrition and water was accepted by competent individuals and by surrogates if such wish had been expressed clearly in writing ahead of time by the patients before they became incompetent.

BABY DOE CASE:

The child referred to as Baby Doe was born with Down's syndrome on April 9, 1982, in Bloomington, Indiana. The child also had a congenital anomaly with tracheoesophageal fistula where there is communication between the breathing passage and food passage, which resulted in constant aspiration and choking. Also, there was a severe mental deficiency. The gynecologist who delivered the baby advised against the operation to repair the fistula, in effect letting it die soon. The parents agreed to a refusal of surgery and also against intravenous feeding. The hospital administrator and other pediatricians opposed this request and went to court. The judge ruled in favor of the parents. The district attorney appealed the case in circuit court and when that failed, they went to the Indiana Supreme Court. The higher court also ruled in favor of the parents. The district attorney filed an appeal to US Supreme Court. The baby died however before the appeal could be heard.

Much wider publicity and outcry sounded in the media against the parents who wanted the child killed in essence. There was much uproar because it was a newborn child and stopping intravenous feeding was seen as a harsher measure. Moreover, it was disclosed that many such babies have been left to die by withdrawing intravenous feeding unofficially in the past. Because of this, the Reagan administration issued a new law requiring hospitals to treat such babies in the future. Hospitals had to place a sign stating that discriminatory failure to feed and care for handicapped babies is prohibited by law and a Baby Doe hotline was set up to report such abuses. When the hotline is called there is an automatic inquiry and investigation. The pediatricians objected to this and the American Academy of Pediatricians went to Federal court to block this rule. The judge ruled for the doctors and agreed that physicians had to decide case by case and the hotline protocol was ill-advised. The Health and Human Services reintroduced the law with some modifications. The second court of appeal again made the law unenforceable. It went to the US Supreme court, which confirmed the lower court decision. During the one year of the law, the Bay Doe Hotline received 1,633 calls. Out of these, 49 cases were investigated, but only 6 babies were suitable for treatment, and out of these, only one baby had survived and the rest died within a few weeks.

Despite these findings, the Federal government issued new regulations in 1985, making it mandatory to provide care for all newborn handicapped babies and any neglect will be treated as child abuse. Intravenous fluids and feeding must be provided to all babies without fail and cannot be withheld unless there is an irreversible comatose state or further treatment is determined to be futile. Assessment of future quality of life is not a valid reason to stop medical treatments regardless of the wishes of the parents. These rules are still in place as of today. The paradoxical legal situation is that fluids and feeding can be withheld to an incompetent adult but not to an incompetent baby.

AID IN DYING:

At a certain point in time, one may wish for a speedy death. There could be any number of reasons behind this wish. There are some options available in the system today.

The first choice is to refuse further medical treatment. Today all of the states in the US allow the right of the otherwise competent patient, to make such a decision, and no explanation is needed. The hospital or doctor may ask the person to sign a statement of refusal to protect themselves against any future claims. If the patient did not sign and walked out, they will just document that the patient signed out against medical advice. The common scenario is to refuse surgery or tests or chemotherapy. An extreme situation is a refusal to take fluids and nutrition.

If the patient is unable to make the decision, the legal guardian or durable power of attorney can make the same decision, if there is a legal document expressing the desires of the patient made while the patient was in a state of sound mind. These documents are called Living Wills and combined with a durable power of attorney the guardian can refuse medical treatment. This scenario is common and legal all over the country.

The next option is Physician-Assisted Suicide (PAS). Here the physician is helping the patient to commit suicide at the request of the patient. This is currently legal in the states of Oregon, California, Washington, Colorado, Hawaii, New Jersey, Vermont, Montana, Maine, and the District of Columbia in the US. It is also legal in other countries such as Canada, the Netherlands, and Belgium. Many strict protocols are to be observed and filed to prevent abuse. The patient must be in sound mind when making the request. Terminal illness and life expectancy less than six months must be verified and documented by two independent physicians. Usually, a high dose of opiates such as morphine or barbiturates is prescribed as a double effect, to reduce pain as well as to reduce respiration. However, the patients must administer the medication by themselves, at their own volition.

The final option is euthanasia. Here the physician is administering the medication instead of the patient self-administering it. This is illegal in all states in the USA, but it is legal in Canada, the Netherlands, and Belgium. The same protocols as a physician-assisted suicide are observed and documented. Euthanasia can be voluntary or involuntary. During voluntary euthanasia, the physician is administering the lethal medicine at the request of the fully competent patient. With involuntary euthanasia, the patient is incompetent, but the physician is still administering the lethal medication considering the best interests of the patient after having studied the medical records, having discussed the situation with the guardians and family, and having determined extreme suffering with imminent death. This is the extreme form of aid in dying and also referred to as "mercy killing".

Despite the laws, it is estimated that doctors do help patients to end their life covertly or indirectly with no records or written documents, in selected cases where they have a direct relationship with the patients or families. The New England Journal of Medicine in March 1999 reported that at least 15,000 physician-assisted deaths are occurring in the USA every year. This is kept as a dirty little secret of medicine.

In my conversations with many individuals, I find most people are not afraid of dying. Those who die are escaping from the sufferings and struggle in this world, and wish to know nothing afterward. They are gone. They always want to die quickly, and painlessly. In the society in which I grew up, it was always a common saying that the wife wants to die first so that she would be dying as a married woman. A widow is looked down upon by the entire family and community. Similarly, all the elderly people in my family always prayed for a fast and quick death without suffering and without becoming a burden on the family. Everyone is afraid of chronic illness and prolonged suffering. They are more afraid of being bedridden with stroke, paralysis, or dementia. They court death and are not afraid of dying.

During my years of internship, residency, and postgraduate training I attended numerous departmental meetings most of them mandatory. The most dreaded meetings were the monthly mortality and morbidity conferences. Death is considered a failure and it is not expected to happen in the hands of doctors. Yet it is a natural event to occur. Even then criticism was leveled at the root causes that led to death. We were guilty of the death based upon the opinions of the seniors and attending. If only you had done this procedure, this test, taken this precaution or intervention it would not have led to this situation. The mortality and morbidity conferences were turned into battlegrounds to tear down the competition and to belittle the enemies, instilling fear and guilt. No sudden death, no unexplained death, and no untreated deaths are acceptable. If it is a slow death over many days or weeks, if everyone has tried any and all treatment measures, then no further questions are asked.

I also think that people in general in India, Africa, and other Asian countries accept death more readily than European and other Western countries do. Maybe it is the culture where one finds answers in Nature and God, instead of finding faults with humans for the death of other humans. Maybe it is the media, that causes unexpected deaths to be blown out of proportion in certain parts of the world, while it is an everyday event in other parts of the world.

Patients, families and doctors, and other health care workers have to work together to have a peaceful and pain-free ending. There has to be a good understanding between them to reach a goal with minimal legalities and formalities. Compassion and kindness are the keywords. Looking at the amount of time commitment and frequency of help, and family members come as first-line helpers. Nurses come next and doctors come as last. It is the words, gestures, body language, and actions that matter most to the patient on the deathbed and not scientific knowledge or medical expertise. Expediting the eventuality should not be seen as suicide or homicide when the days are numbered and pain control and reducing suffering are the most desired outcomes. The doctor should be willing to certify the cause of death as the underlying disease, nurses should be willing to provide comfort measures and pain control, the family should be willing to provide personal touches on caring. The soul should be able to depart with happiness and bliss.

Chapter 24

DYING WITH DIGNITY

Where would you like to die?

When asked, nine out of ten would like to die in their home, in their familiar surroundings, in their bed, with their family, spouse, and children nearby in peace and comfort. There is no doubt this is the best way, but only a fortunate four out of ten can achieve it. The rest are forced to die in the hospital, or nursing home, or extended care facilities. The least fortunate ones die in the streets or battlefields or unknown gutters or similar forsaken places.

Everyone would agree that a hospital is not a good place to die with dignity. Too many regulations, too many interruptions, changes of personnel, formal attitudes, legalities, blood tests, intravenous fluids, tubes and catheters, forceful treatments, an inability to sleep due to noise, lights, and nursing care, and high costs are just some of the issues. Nursing homes and long-term care facilities are for those who do not have families or families who cannot or will not take care of them.

The best place to die in dignity is in your own home, in your bed, cared for by your spouse or other family members. They may engage a nursing aid to give personal care such as washing or bathing, but the family member is always there for you.

Unfortunately, one-fifth of Americans die in the hospital ICU, and many more get shuttled through the hospital in the last few months of their lives. We tend to take them to the hospital when they become acutely ill. We want to make sure we are not neglecting them, we want to correct any acute correctable problems, and we want to provide emergency care. Sad to say, certain medical treatments can easily be referred to as being aggressive or even unnecessary. They are done either out of fear or ignorance or pure greed to make money. Examples of such situations are inserting a pacemaker or defibrillator on a 90 plus-year-old terminally ill patient with limited life expectancy, or taking a similar person for hemodialysis. Advanced medicine is capable of prolonging life without any meaning or quality. It is up to the family and family doctor, to avoid hospitalization of a terminally ill person. This requires planning and getting the all individuals on the same page.

Studies done in the past have shown that a large number of patients endured painful and prolonged deaths due to unjustified heroic life-supporting treatments with no objective or goal. Pulling the plug was a taboo and was done quietly with unspoken words. Fear of many people was not the death itself, but that they might die after a prolonged period of agony, pain, and suffering from an inability to communicate with their loved ones on the last few days of their life.

Several other people are forced into long-term care facilities or adult living facilities. Their children may be successful and they may be wealthy, but they do not have the time or interest, or opportunity to care for their elderly parents. Modern societal living has changed the joint family system where the elderly are easily taken care of by the working younger people. Not anymore, the children are in foreign countries or faraway cities, busy with their affairs. The empty nesters are living in extended care facilities, talking about their children since they have no other choice.

Pain Management: One of the main types of suffering is from pain. Everyone wants to die without pain or suffering, but only about half are fortunate to have pain controlled. The only humane act is to relieve the pain of a terminally ill person. Pain can be due to fractures, nerve compressions, tumor growths, soft tissue infections, musculoskeletal problems, degenerative disorders, or head and neck disorders. Some of them are in constant pain. The only time when they do not have pain is when they are sleeping. They need adequate pain medications in doses high enough to control the pain. Dying in dignity requires an understanding of physician and family who will see to it that they do not suffer from unnecessary pain. A morphine pump or a PCA (patient-controlled analgesia) would be a valuable adjunct. Morphine is a very useful drug in controlling pain for the terminally ill. The word morphine is derived from Morpheus, the Greek God of dreams, one of the sons of Somnus, the God of Sleep.

Pain management has become a hot topic recently because of opioid addiction leading to over 70,000 deaths a year in the US. Only 20 years ago, it was felt that patients were not getting adequate pain control, and Congress approved laws to encourage pain control. Specialties evolved purely on pain management with several of the anesthesiologists branching off into this field. They would do epidurals, various nerve blocks, insert morphine pumps, and give out prescriptions. Many pain pill mills evolved prescribing oral painkillers such as oxycontin. Later they evolved into the use of fentanyl and other injectable medications. Now, this has gone overboard with the federal government beginning to crack down on pain managers. The reality is that there needs to be a happy medium. Those who are terminally ill and having chronic pain syndromes must be able to get pain medications as needed to keep them comfortable. It is unfair to withhold pain medications from them in the name of addiction possibility. Acute pain related to infections, surgery, trauma must also get adequate pain control in times of need. There is no need to make these patients suffer or be tortured.

Sleep management: Another suffering is the inability to sleep and agitation. This can be due to neurological or metabolic problems. Anxiety and stress can take over and depression can set in. These patients need proper amounts of sedation and relaxants. Barbiturates are the most useful here. A lack of sleep causes more stress, irritability, and medical and mental problems. Over 40% of the population has insomnia. Fear of suicide and addiction once again leads to inadequate prescriptions for sleep management. During sleep hours, the brain gets much-required rest, it washes off toxins built up, new neurons sprout and the brain regenerates. All of us notice that after a night of good sleep we feel refreshed and energized. After a night of poor sleep, we feel tired, depressed, and listless, irritable, and angry.

Empathy: Words of empathy, kindness, and caring are extremely appreciated by the terminally ill. It is not uncommon for them to be hated by some caregivers or family members as a burden or a chore. The last thing the dying person wants to hear is being blamed and feeling neglected. Words can be harsh and hurting. The dying person wants to die as quickly and as peacefully as possible.

Many patients have neurological disorders, dementia, or Alzheimer's disease. Toxicity of chemicals accumulating in the blood from kidney or liver diseases can affect the brain function. These patients may be agitated, irrational, forgetful, or even violent due to confusion. In hospitals and nursing homes, nurses like to restrain patients who are likely to be agitated or likely to fall. They want to protect them from falling from the bed or from pulling out tubes and catheters. However, restraining is bad. It is better to sedate them. It is proven by animal experiments that restraining causes ulcers to develop in the stomach and causes further aggravation and stress.

When first diagnosed with an incurable condition or cancer, there are several stages in the acceptance of a terminal illness and in the process of dying. These stages include an initial denial that leads to anger, then a stage of bargaining, and then a stage of depression, and finally a stage of acceptance. People may react differently to these stages. Some may stay in one stage for longer than others, some may skip some stages and some may not reach the final stage of acceptance at all. We, humans, are different from each other.

There is a difference between prolonging life versus relieving suffering when it comes to the care of the dying. Dying with dignity means dying in comfort, both physically and emotionally. Mere prolongation of life with continued daily suffering from pain, sleeplessness, and discomfort is not worthwhile. This does not mean that one should stop nutrition and fluids or simple medical treatments either. It would be necessary to refuse certain types of medical treatments while continuing common-sense treatments, particularly pain medications, sedatives, and sleeping aids.

Thich Nhat Hanh is a celebrated Buddhist monk from Vietnam, described as one of the most influential spiritual leaders of our times, and is now 92 years old. After a venerable life in various countries, he is now at a villa outside Hue, in Vietnam, as a terminally ill person. He refuses all modern medicines and treatments, waiting for liberation. Devotees and diplomats and even heads of States came to visit him for a last glimpse. He is referred to as the Father of Mindfulness, a modern-day form of meditation and stress relief tactics. He has authored over 70 books, and Miracle of Mindfulness is a favored teaching. His teaching is that you do not have to go to extreme steps and mountaintops to seek spirituality. You can find it in simple things, in your breath, in your everyday activity, mixing it up with joy and compassion. This became very appealing to Westerners seeking spirituality without religion, leading to an entire mindfulness movement. Today, 35% of companies incorporate mindfulness in their workplace, and it has become a 1.1 billion dollar industry, with 2500 meditation centers, books, apps, and online courses. Nhat Hanh is waiting quietly for his "transition" on the grounds of a 19th century Tu Hieu Pagoda Buddhist temple.

Ultimately the individual himself or herself also has to take moral responsibility for passing with peace and comfort. It should be seen as the passage pre-destined, not to be seen as a struggle and fight for a few more days. With proper planning, with the help of friends and family, and with the help of doctors and nurses, one can make it easy for oneself as well as for others. There should be acceptance without crying or sadness, with a celebration of life.

It appears as though the entire medical system or health care field is geared to take care of illnesses, sickness, injuries, accidents, and other acute events. Much less emphasis is given to providing wellbeing, preventative care, and long term care. Old age and related maintenance issues are not attractive to the vast majority of doctors. The hospitals spend a huge amount of resources and expenses on prolonging the last few days or weeks of life, knowing well in advance that such a prolongation of life is only for a short time, which may be only days or weeks. The last three months of a person's life have become the most expensive. Even if they survive and go home, they return to die within a short period. There is an innate refusal to accept the eventuality of death. We consider success as measured by discharge from the hospital alive, not by the quality of life afterward. In her book Knocking on Heaven's Door, Katy Butler asks when does death cease being a curse and become a blessing? Where is the line between saving life and prolong dying? When is the right time to say to a doctor "let my loved one go" The medical system is a broken and morally-adrift labyrinth with amazing advances in therapy and tangled webs of technology along with legal protocols interplaying with business interests and financial considerations.

Pacemakers and defibrillators (AICD) can be deactivated in an otherwise terminally ill patient if that is the only device that is keeping them alive. Experts from the American Heart Association and American College of Cardiology have written statements that disabling a pacemaker or defibrillator is neither physician-assisted suicide nor euthanasia. The patient or durable power attorney has a legal and moral right to request such deactivation. (Lampert, Rachel et al. HRS Expert consensus statement on management of cardiovascular implantable electronic devices in patients nearing the end of life or requesting withdrawal of therapy- Heart Rhythm, July 2010).

For the past several years there is a better recognition of palliative care, pain management, hospice care, physiotherapy, and geriatric care. These topics should be taught to all medical students. Only a few physicians opt for practice in these fields as their chosen specialty. The most important element required here is compassion and kindness and not medicine or surgery. However, these ideals are quickly lost in the practice of medical science and in the quest to make money. There is also job satisfaction when an impossible and difficult clinical challenge is met with the latest device or technology as compared to just talking to an old person and making sure he or she is walking, peeing, and pooping. While doctors can do only so much, the burden is transferred to nurses. The most important person who can do the most is a family member.

Chapter 25

EUTHANASIA

This is a true story of euthanasia that was carried out four years ago, but later on was charged as first-degree murder. (Tampa Bay Times, March 6, 2019). An 85-year-old male had told his two daughters that he does not wish to be in a nursing home or extended care facility during his last days. He also had dementia and other age-related medical problems. The daughters gave him heavy alcohol with sleeping pills and he fell asleep on the couch. They thought he would die, but he lived. Then they tried to smother him with a pillow, but he kept on breathing. Then they held him by force and stuffed clothes into his mouth and pinched his nose. He finally died. Afterward, they removed all evidence and called paramedics by calling 911. He was certified as having died of natural age-related problems.

Four years later both the sisters became romantically involved with the same man. They confessed to the man about how they had killed their father. He tape-recorded the conversation and handed it over to the police. The sheriff's office reopened the case and upon questioning the sisters, they both confessed to the crime. They had gotten away with the euthanasia, but they spilled the beans four years later. Now the sisters are facing a court sentence.

The word euthanasia is derived from Greek- 'EU' meaning 'good' and 'Thanatos' meaning death, meaning good death. Currently, it means inducing death out of kindness like shooting a disabled horse. It means inducing death, not necessarily at the request of the patient, because one takes pity on the incurability and suffering by the patient. Referred to as mercy killing. The decision to induce death can be taken by the doctor, family, or the patient. Supporters call it a civil right or self-determination. Opponents call it murder or mercy killing and link it with the Holocaust. Euthanasia involves intentional termination of life whether the patient requests for the same or not. The physician decides it, taking into consideration what is best for the patient. The family may request the termination of life or the patient may also request help. In any case, the physician, without active participation by the patient induces termination of life.

Euthanasia can be passive euthanasia or active euthanasia. In passive euthanasia, one is letting the person die with no further medical treatment or life support. It is a more painful and prolonged course that includes measures such as stopping tube feedings, disconnecting the respirator, and so forth. In the active form of euthanasia, one is administering medications to expedite death. This could be in the form of excessive morphine or barbiturates or helium inhalation. Active euthanasia can be voluntary, when requested by the patient or involuntary when unrequested by the patient (often when a patient is incompetent or unable to make decisions, but requested by the family, power of attorney, or caregiver).

Euthanasia is not permitted in any of the states in the US. It is possible in certain European countries such as Belgium, Holland, and Switzerland. It is also legal in Canada. In-State of Washington, in 1991 a proposal to permit euthanasia reached the ballot, but it was voted out. The public wanted many safeguards against abuse of the opportunity.

During the Second World War, Hitler's Nazi Germany made euthanasia into a state of horror. The government had a program to eliminate all those who were "unworthy of life". It started with mentally disabled children, then expanded to mentally or physically challenged adults. Subsequently, it also expanded to include Jews and minorities. Many medical and surgical researches were done based on this. The rationale was partly economic, partly political. There was no point in having all those sick ones to be cared for with Germany's tight budget. It was seen as the right thing to get rid of socially and religiously "unwanted" individuals so that only the good locals needed to breed. Many German physicians willingly participated in it as the right thing to do.

JACK KEVORKIAN: He was a retired pathologist from Michigan. Dr. Jack Kevorkian was the major proponent of physician-assisted suicide. He became aggressive to the extent of promoting euthanasia, which was difficult for society to accept. He brought major attention to the public about the right to die, physician-assisted suicide, and euthanasia as never before.

He claimed to have assisted in over 150 suicides, daring the State of Michigan to prosecute him. During the 1980s and 1990's he was a well-known figure, people calling him Dr. Death and Jack the Dripper.

He had invented a homemade machine made out of scrap metal, that will allow the patient to self-inject a lethal dose of medication. News magazines called it a "mercitron". He had not examined nor taken care of these patients. They came to him seeking assistance in dying. He had not looked at their case histories or talked to their doctors. Some of the cases had undergone an autopsy, which failed to reveal a life-threatening, or terminal illness. However, he did publicize these events, videotaped them, and created a huge wave of awareness.

His license to practice medicine was revoked. Charges against him were successfully defended. When he could not prescribe or obtain lethal drugs, he tried to use carbon monoxide, the patients initiated steps of which.

On September 17, 1998, he injected a lethal dose of narcotics into a 52-year-old man with amyotrophic lateral sclerosis (ALS) at his request and with his family's permission. He videotaped the event and sent it to CBS television to broadcast it in "60 minutes" for the sake of national publicity. This was obviously a mercy killing, and the murder trial was brought against him. Kevorkian wanted to defend the case by himself, which was rambling. The jury found him guilty of second-degree murder and the use of unauthorized narcotics. He was sentenced to a 10- 25 years prison sentence.

Chapter 26

PHYSICIAN ASSISTED SUICIDE

Many ancient societies have accepted suicide and physician-assisted suicide as an honorable thing to do. Ancient Greeks have not only accepted suicide but also have requested help from the government to do so. Suicide on the war field was considered preferable and righteous rather than being captured as a slave in Japan and India. Womenfolk committed suicide by poison or self-immolation rather than being raped or abused during war times. The elderly, sick, and disabled wanted to end their lives rather than prolong suffering.

Opposition to suicide in any form began to take effect with the progress of religions. Hippocrates in his oath to physicians expressly forbids them to give drugs that will expedite the death of the patients even if they so request. Christianity, Islam as well as Judaism condemned suicide. It was not the right of humans to take lives given by the Gods and only God is allowed to take that life back.

In physician-assisted suicide, the patient is requesting to exit out due to the suffering and takes an active role in inducing the death with the help of the physician. It is slightly different from euthanasia as described previously.

It is a movement of the "right to choose to die", which is always in conflict with the "right to live". The right to die, group, wants individual freedom, not only to die but also to die when they want and how they want. They feel that competent adults with a terminal illness or less than six months to live should have a right to refuse further medical treatment and be able to receive help from a physician and medical community to end their lives.

The "right to live movement" feels that it is the state's responsibility to protect life and preserve it. They do not want abuses by physicians, nurses, or patients to cause unnecessary deaths. It is God who gave them life and it is up to God to decide when and how to end it.

Hemlock Society and supporters provided a forum to discuss the auto-euthanasia in justifiable cases. Derek Humphrey started the Hemlock Society in the USA in 1980. He helped his first wife who was suffering from incurable cancer to commit suicide and published a book on this, "*Jean's Way: A Love Story*". The name Hemlock is derived from a poisonous root plant, which was used in ancient times in Greece and Rome to commit suicide. The society supports the principle of ending a person's own life when faced with a terminal illness, suffering, and pain. It has various publications, and local chapters and provides general help through physicians and without breaking the law. It has two books, "*Let me die before I wake*" and "*Final Exit*". There were over seventy local chapters and over 40,000 members as of 1992. In the year of 2003, it changed its name to End-of-Life Choices, as a nonprofit organization. It also developed two special programs: Caring Friends Program and the Patient Advocacy Program. They provide a full range of advice, information, and options for end of life management including physician aided suicide, but without getting involved in direct services or physical assistance, staying within the legal boundaries. They are advocacy groups for end-of-life choices including euthanasia and provide literature and information to those who request. They will ensure that the patient's documented instructions are followed and honored.

Compassion in Dying is another activist organization in Oregon since 1993. They advise patients on all options including high dose pain medications and terminal sedation.

They helped to win court rulings on allowing pain medication during the end of life care.

In 2004, the above two organizations, End of Life Choices and Compassion in Dying merged to form a new entity called Compassion and Choices. In the same year, another group by the name Final Exit Network was formed, which offers a personal guide to members only.

Physician-Assisted Suicide is legal in the states of Oregon, California, Colorado, Washington, Hawaii, New Jersey, Vermont, Montana, Maine, and the District of Columbia in the US. Oregon law on Physician-Assisted Suicide became effective in 1997. Several safeguards were set up to avoid mistakes or abuse.

The patient must be 18 years and must be an Oregon resident for at least six months.

The patient must submit a written request with two witnesses, and two additional verbal witnessed confirmations on two separate days fifteen days apart and these must be documented.

Two independent physicians must attest that the patient is terminally ill with less than six months to live.

Physicians must attest that patient is in sound mind and judgment and capable of making their own independent decisions.

The patient must be able to self-administer the medications. The physician must document the diagnosis, prognosis, and prescriptions given and consumed. The physician must report about the case and outcome to Oregon Public Health Service. The medication given most commonly were barbiturates.

On the international scene, physician-assisted suicide is legal in the Netherlands, Belgium, and Switzerland. They are also accepted in Australia and Canada. In many of the third world countries and Asian countries, all rules and regulations are loose and murky. Physicians have great freedom and their actions are mostly unchallenged by society. Record keeping and data reliability are poor.

Those who support the "right to die" movement believe that competent adults who have less than six months to live have the right to make self-determination to end their suffering and misery. They know that they have an incurable and serious illness such as advanced cancer or degenerative disorders with no hope. They want to reduce their pain and suffering and being a burden to their caregivers. They are asking not only to stop life-sustaining treatments but also to request their physicians to help them to end the misery.

The right to refuse treatment as well as the right to stop life-sustaining measures is now legal across the US if it is requested by competent patients or by the durable power of attorneys with written advance directives by the patient made at the time of sound frame of mind, such as a Living Will.

Those who oppose the movement feel it is the State's duty is to preserve and prolong life and no individual has a right to shorten it under any conditions. Suicide is a crime and any form of intentional termination of life is also a crime. They also fear that it will be abused similar to abortion rights and many people will be killed. The elderly and mentally disabled will be eliminated for the gains of the family members.

In the fourth century BC, Greek physician Hippocrates established a set of promises to be made by the physicians called the Hippocrates Oath, which is a pledge to practice good medicine. In it, one of the pledges is "I will not give a deadly drug to anybody if asked for it, nor will I make a suggestion to that effect". Ironically enough in 399 BC, the philosopher Socrates was asked to drink the poison of hemlock as a penalty for corrupting the minds of youth in Greece.

There is reason to believe that under certain circumstances physicians are assisting in suicide without documentation on personal requests from time to time. Many of these take place as terminal sedation or withdrawal of treatment under their guidance which is kept as a secret to avoid legal issues. There are no accurate data on this since it is undisclosed, but various prior surveys estimate about 15,000 such physician-assisted deaths occur each year in the US.

What are the actual modalities used to hasten the death? One obvious measure is to withhold tube feeding including water and nutrients until the person becomes dehydrated and starvation occurs. This takes a few days of agony. Another method is to give increasing dosages of barbiturates, allowing the person to go into a deep sleep. Giving an increasing dosage of morphine helps to relieve pain and allows the person to sleep.

The use of helium gas with a tight mask is useful to expedite death within a few minutes. The person becomes anoxic with no oxygen entering the system, while exhalation of carbon dioxide allows freedom from thrashing or agitation. Brain death occurs within four minutes when there is no oxygen going into the brain. When someone is suffocated by such methods as strangulation or a pillow over the face or by hanging, there is a good amount of thrashing, jerking, and fighting because of difficulty in exhaling carbon dioxide and not because of lack of oxygen. The advantages of using helium are many. Barbiturates need a prescription that is becoming harder and harder to obtain in lethal doses. One will have to accumulate the drug in small quantities over a period of time, and one needs to find a sympathetic and cooperative doctor. Many protocols are to be observed if it becomes known that there is physician-assisted suicide behind the motif. Helium does not need a prescription; one can go to a party store and get a tank of helium to blow up balloons. The death is fast and quick in four minutes compared to several hours with other modalities. It is painless and struggle-free because you are exhaling carbon dioxide while inhaling helium. It does need however a helpful family to carry it out and a helpful doctor who will issue a death certificate based on the underlying disease. Helium is colorless and odorless and non-inflammable and non-explosive. There are detailed instructions available as to how to use the helium, using a plastic bag or a collapsible large plastic tent with Velcro strapping around the neck and over the head with a tube inserted inside or using a very tight-fitting facemask with no leakage as they use in CPAP

(Continuous positive airway pressure) for sleep apnea. The idea is to inhale helium instead of oxygen or room air and exhale carbon dioxide freely without any obstruction as it is the accumulation of carbon dioxide in the body that causes the choking sensation with resultant agitation, thrashing, and fighting.

Doctors can write orders at the request of the patient or family members, based on the documented Living Will and medical proxy, to facilitate the end of life care in certain ways. Such an order could be a DNR (Do Not Resuscitate) or CMO (Comfort Measures Only) or referral to Hospice care. Each of these has different meanings and protocols. A DNR order prevents calling a "code" when there is a cardiac arrest. When a "code" is called in the hospital, a bunch of doctors and nurses rush to the bedside, pump the chest, intubate the airway and connect to a respirator, and give various medications to keep the patient alive and transfer the patient to the intensive care unit. Hence it is better not to call the code and this is where the DNR order comes in handy. However, during the DNR status, one agrees to take normal medications, nutrition, antibiotics, physiotherapy, and even surgery.

A question comes up about pacemakers and defibrillators. Should one insert these devices in certain patients at all? Many patients in the nursing home who have no quality of life, non-ambulating, and even with a Living Will are transferred to a hospital emergency room due to slow heartbeat or low blood pressure, or irregular heartbeat. They are often treated with emergency insertion of pacemakers. No one wants to stop the treatment either due to legal reasons, or monetary reasons, or moral issues. Such expensive treatments simply prolong the agony of a dying person.

Another moral and ethical question asked is about the deactivation of pacemakers and defibrillators on a living person. The defibrillators are routinely deactivated before any surgery and anesthesia and then reactivated later. Many patients are brain dead, but the heart is kept beating only because of the pacemaker. All dead persons will show a pacemaker rhythm on the cardiogram until it is turned off. Hospital nurses do this step almost routinely once the person is declared dead. If one deactivates a pacemaker on an elderly terminally patient to hasten the death, can it be interpreted as physician-assisted suicide or euthanasia? What are the legal implications here? Both the American College of Cardiology and the American Heart Association have clear statements that deactivating a functioning pacemaker or defibrillator is not physician-assisted suicide and that it is not euthanasia. It is a medical decision by the doctor based on facts on hand.

An Order for Comfort Measures Only (CMO) goes one step further than DNR orders. Here the patient or family has requested only minimal treatment with the understanding that death is imminent, and does not want any treatments except those medications and measures to keep the patient comfortable and pain-free. Usually, an intravenous line is maintained for fluids and sedatives, and pain medications. No antibiotics are given and no further tests or aggressive treatments are done. Nutrition may or may not be provided but without the use of a feeding tube.

Everyone over the age of 18 should realize how important it is to have a Living Will and a signed medical proxy. Everyone also needs to know their rights; the right to get pain relief, the right to change doctors, the right to question medical treatments, the right to refuse treatment, the right to refuse tube feedings, the right to refuse CPR, and life support. Every patient has the right to decide and not the society or courts to decide one's health care and control over their own body. Unfortunately, certain religious minorities and courts stand on the side of the right to life confusing the issues of desires for the terminally ill with other forms of termination of life.

The Canadian Supreme court decriminalized physician assistance for patients suffering from grievous illness and irremediable conditions to hasten their death in the year 2015. The following year the Canadian government passed legislation to permit physician-assisted suicide (where prescriptions can be given to a patient who takes it voluntarily) and for voluntary euthanasia (where the medication to terminate life is administered by the physician, at the request of the patient).

Section-7- Beginning of life

Chapter 27

GENETICS

We need to go to the beginning of life to understand the end of life. Who created life on this planet, when was it created, and how was it done? When and how were the humans created?

The Bible says there was chaos in the beginning. Then God created the earth, and then all the animals, plants, and finally, he created man and woman. There is truth in this. Hinduism thinks there was a deluge and then God created life from the ocean. There is truth in this too. Japanese and ancient tribal Indians worshipped the Sun God as the source. There is truth in this as well. Modern-day scientists have theories but no clear answer. Life is estimated to have begun on earth about 3.5 billion years ago, through a natural process by which inorganic chemicals gave way to primitive living factors with the help of water, hydrogen, lightning, and the sun. Yet still, no one can create new lives in a laboratory out of these chemicals to this date.

If there is a miracle in the world it is the birth of a new person. Imagine the single cell called zygote after fertilization of the ovum by the sperm. This one cell carries with it all the codes and mysteries to convert the subsequent cells into lungs, heart, ears, nose, and such to make a complete human body. Can anyone believe that the entire mango tree came out of one small tiny seed? How were the codes installed in them? Could just a drop of chemical compounds that made life happen?

The second miracle is death when all activity is shut off on short notice, just like turning the light switch off. What happens to that glob of a chemical compound? Why does it misbehave and stop working? Both birth and death have many unanswered questions.

The field of molecular genetics includes the physical and chemical structure of the genes, DNA (Deoxyribonucleic acid), and its expressions. Primary organisms like bacteria and ameba do not have a nucleus inside their cells and the DNA is loosely floating around inside the cell membrane. They are called Prokaryotes. When the time comes for them to duplicate, the DNA copies itself through a process of replication and the cell divides into two. The original and offspring are identical in all aspects. We also call this process mitosis. There are billions and billions of bacteria all around us and we live with them.

Further developed species including humans have a well-defined nucleus inside the cell called Eukaryotes. Their DNA strands are held inside the nucleus. Their reproduction is through a complicated process called recombination. The male and female cells come together, with a mix and match of the two different DNA strands that create a completely new genetic offspring. The parents and offspring will have similarities, but they are completely different from their parents. This process is called meiosis.

DNA is a double helix strand, that replicates itself through a process of copying the DNA accurately. These strands exist in the form of chromosomes. Both strands are replicated after unraveling the helix. DNA is made of millions of nucleotides held together in the strands. The nucleotides are made of deoxyribose, one of the bases of adenine, guanine, thymine, or cytosine, (A G T C), and three phosphates. Replication occurs with help of several enzymes, such as helicase that opens up the helix, gyrase that prevents the helix from making knots, and telomerase that replicates the ends of chromosomes, and other enzymes that help in the process. "A" is always paired with "T" and "G" is always paired with "C", thus ensuring the code is copied exactly when DNA reproduces itself. DNA is life. Every organism on the planet relies on DNA to store genetic information and transmit it from generation to generation. The coded information inside a chromosome is similar to the microchip of a computer, holding information equal to a large library.

RNA (ribonucleic acid) is like a brother of DNA and carries the messages of DNA out of the nucleus into the cell cytoplasm. RNA is single-stranded. DNA provides the template and the RNA takes it to make the proteins or polypeptides. In other words, life is just a group of chemicals held together.

About 99.9% of the 6 billion steps in the double helix staircase of DNA are the same for all humans. This is what differentiates humans from other species. The remaining 0.1% of the molecules in the DNA are determining the individuals of who each of us becomes, the differences in our looks, behavior, and personality. There is some influence from the environment, society, and family in which a person grows, but the DNA essentially determines the nature of the person. It is possible to map out differences between DNA by a new technology called SNP chips, which stands for Single Nucleotide Polymorphism.

Probably life began on planet earth about 3.5 billion years ago, when the biological molecules of proteins, nucleic acids, and energy particles came together to create the micro-organisms. Progressively they expanded by mutations and then meiosis. Possibly Darwin's theory of evolution has valid explanations with the natural selection and survival of the fittest. However, the fact remains that every cell has the DNA and RNA molecules made of chemicals that come together.

The first single-cell initially carried genetic instructions to make any type of cell subsequently. After some time, they lose the ability to create new genes, and aging occurs. Initially, they lose the ability to make all kinds of cells but can reproduce the same type of cell. Then they die gradually and completely, as the telomeres cannot stick together anymore. Yet why are they unable to sustain it? What happened to the glob of chemical that was held together? If we can find the answer, we can also stop aging and look towards further longevity. Scientists have been able to identify eight genes that influence aging.

Gene therapy has opened up new boundaries in treating medical problems. Treatment by replacing faulty genes with healthy ones offers the potential for curing many diseases like hemophilia and muscular dystrophy. According to a report from the drug industry, nearly 300 gene therapies are under development to treat over 100 diseases. Billions of dollars are at stake here. For example, the Roche Company agreed to buy a start-up by name Spark Therapeutics for one and a half times its market value. They were approved to market a drug called Luxturna that treats a rare hereditary condition that causes blindness. The price tag for the drug is $850,000 for one treatment. Million-dollar drugs are not unforeseen in the future. Novartis is developing gene therapy called Zolgensma for spinal muscular dystrophy to be available in five years but at a cost of over one million dollars per patient. Other approved gene therapies are Kymriah (Novartis) and Yescarta (Gilead sciences) both for the treatment of leukemia.

There are two types of gene therapy. One is called replacement gene therapy and the other is called gene-editing therapy. In the replacement therapy, a neutered virus carrying a new gene is made to bind with the cell membrane of the host. The virus breaks down and allows the new gene to be injected into the cell nucleus and the cell functions in a new way.

Gene editing uses the CRISPR-CAS 9 technique. (Clustered Regularly Interspaced Short Palindromic Repeats) A synthetic guide RNA is used to find the target DNA strand. The RNA travels with an enzyme called CAS9. This enzyme cuts off the DNA strand that is defective and replaces it with a healthy one.

Efforts are underway to manipulate the DNA in such a way to create designer babies. It is futuristic and science fiction. Yet someday it will be possible to create life. So far, it remains a mystery, a miracle, and an impossible dream. Genes and DNA are the answers for life, aging, and eventual death.

Chapter-28

STEM CELLS

In the movie, "Island" (2005), a hidden research farm is shown, where cloned babies are grown and kept for future use by the millionaire owners, for their personal needs. When the time comes, they would harvest the required body part from the cloned babies to replace their own worn-out or diseased body part by transplantation. A similar theme is in the movie "Never Let Me Go" (2010), where clones are grown for the harvesting of their body parts.

There are many horror stories and claims of aborted baby's parts being used to grow new organs, which may not be false. During Nazi rule in Germany live human experimentations took place in various biomedical unethical conduct. For example, it was decided by the government to get rid of undesirable and unwanted people from society by eliminating them. In Japan from 1945 to 1990 about 25,000 people were forced to undergo mandatory sterilization since they were undesirable citizens to have children. It included again mentally and physically handicapped people. The government apologized publicly in 2019 and gave them compensation belatedly.

Another human experimentation was in the USA, when in 1932 a research institute in Tuskegee, Alabama enrolled 600 poor black males and infected 400 of them with syphilis to study the progression of the disease. They were monitored for 40 years and the study was stopped in 1972 after huge public outcry. Even though penicillin was available to cure them, they were never treated and lied to. Since then stricter enforcement laws against biological experimentations on humans have been put in place.

Stem cells are special cells that can become any type of cell or grow to an unlimited level. This ability is called plasticity. The fertilized human egg with early embryonic cells also known as blastomeres has the highest degree of plasticity. We know that they can create an entire body consisting of multiple organs by dividing and differentiating. These are called totipotent or pluripotent cells. As the organ grows, the plasticity of the cells decreases. Afterward, they can only multiply as multipotent cells or create the same type of cells.

Stem cells are thus divided into two broad categories-Pluripotent and multipotent. Pluripotent cells are also referred to as Embryonic Stem Cells, (ESC), and can become any type of cell whereas multipotent cells, also known as Adult Stem Cells can only make lineages. The third category is called Induced Pluripotent stem cells (iPSC), which are reprogramed multipotent cells to make them behave like pluripotent cells, first described by Yamanaka and Thomson in 2007 in independent studies. Such technology holds the highest research potential for the future.

The current emphasis is on stem cells in the field of regenerative medicine. With the advent of reprogramming technology, a new class of stem cells called Induced Pluripotent Stem Cells can be made, from multipotent cells. These research developments have given new modalities for treating various disorders. Stem cells can be isolated from embryos, umbilical cord, or from adult tissues. When cultured correctly the stem cells can be made to learn to cure diseases. Such stem cell research is being done to cure spinal cord problems, Alzheimer's disease, heart diseases, and certain cancers.

If stem cells can replace worn-out red blood cells and white blood cells, they may be able to repair other worn-out organs such as the heart and lung or brain. Angiogenesis to create new blood vessels inside organs to regrow the tissue is being tried.

Stem cells are taken from bone marrow, often called bone marrow transplantation, and has been used to treat leukemia and lymphomas, and metastatic cancers. The patient is given a high dose of chemotherapy and radiation therapy, which destroys the patient's bone marrow. Then the new bone marrow is infused to reestablish the system.

Stem cells can be harvested from newborn babies or aborted babies, from the umbilical cord blood or bone marrow. There is also a pathway to harvest them from peripheral blood after giving a course of growth cell promoting medication. The growth factor GCSF (Granulocyte-colony Stimulating Factor) is given for 4 or 5 days, and then the blood is drawn and sent through a process of apheresis to collect the stem cells from the rest of the components.

Steady new discoveries and research in the field of stem cell therapy and medical science are looking at new frontiers. There is a report on in utero treatment of alpha thalassemia by injecting stem cells into the umbilical vein and correcting congenital anomalies at the University of California, San Francisco. A Japanese team headed by Shinya Yamanaka from Kyoto University showed the ability to generate stem cells from skin cells, avoiding the need to get embryonic stem cells from fetal tissues, by creating Induced Pluripotent stem cells (iPS). They can be coaxed to develop into different organs such as neural cells, heart muscle, or pancreatic cells. Stem cells can lead to replacing dead or ailing cells with new regenerating cells, thus making it possible for cells instead of drugs to treat diseases.

The study of stem cells leads us to discuss when life actually begins. Is it already alive in the male sperm and female ovum and they just made a reconfiguration after fertilization? Or is it the fertilized ovum with a single cell containing millions of genetic information, like a microchip holding thousands of pages of books that describe you as a person who is going to develop out that single cell? If so when did the soul and body begin to function as "you"? It came together at that moment of conception. The chemical complexes and physical structure that became the body was given the personality of 'you' by the soul, similar to the software that makes the hardware of the computer to do wonders. In the same way after death, the physical structure made of chemical complexes can wear off but the soul can live. The software can be inserted into other hardware and make it compute again.

One of the new developments in stem cell research is in what is called a Crispr-Cas9 system, introduced in 2012. It is a way of editing the gene. It consists of two parts- an RNA guide, which can help to target a specific location on a genome, and the Cas9 protein, which acts as molecular scissors. Thus they can edit the DNA of sperms, eggs, and embryos, implementing changes that can be passed down to future generations.

In 1987 scientists observed that some bacteria have the Crisper-Cas9 gene that helps them to defend against invading viruses. Australian scientists have been working on this technology for several years and have used it in different animals and birds. They are able to bring back extinct species. They feel it is not far from the future when designer babies can be made with excellence in sports, arts, or intelligence. It is also quite possible to increase longevity for an uncertain number of years and make immortality possible. It is possible to control mosquitos' genes to reduce transmission of illnesses, improve agricultural products, and cure illnesses such as cystic fibrosis, sickle cell anemia.

News media reported on November 27, 2018, that a Chinese scientist had produced a genetically edited newborn human twin babies. 'He Jiankui' of Southern University of Science and Technology of China said he altered the DNA of twin girls to help them resist HIV infection. Initially, an embryologist fertilized the mother's egg with the sperm of the father. Immediately thereafter an enzyme was introduced inside the newly formed embryo, which altered its gene, and then the modified developing embryo was implanted into the mother's womb. The newborn baby had the modified gene. There is no independent confirmation of this feat, and no details were disclosed to other peer review group. He performed the feat to help HIV infected parents have uninfected children. He also wanted to make China a pioneer country in gene technology.

DNA editing is currently banned in the US, and over 100 scientists across the globe immediately denounced the effort by Mr. He. Moreover, Mr. He reported this on YouTube as a video instead of presenting it in scientific journals or conferences. The Chinese government also penalized him for unauthorized gene editing in newborn children.

Gene editing is an uncertain process, complicated and can have many unexpected side effects. Most bioethicists and geneticists have expressed serious concern and reservations on using this in animals and particularly in humans. The attempt to create leaner rabbits caused their tongues to become large, pigs developed extra vertebrae, and gene-edited calves died prematurely. Many things about gene editing, DNA modification, and after-effects are still unknown. Some benefits are touted such as cattle without horns, making the meat processing easier, and gene-edited wool from Merino sheep.

Gene therapy is a new frontier in treating certain medical conditions in adults. Genes are attached to innocuous viruses and infused. These viruses insert the gene into the cells correcting the dysfunction. Such revolutionary therapy is used in cancer treatment, using Chimeric Antigen Receptor T cells (CART). Treated T cells are infused back into the body to destroy abnormal B cells. The treatment is effective in patients with certain types of leukemia and lymphomas.

Platelet Rich Plasma (PRP) treatment: This modality of treatment has some elements of self-healing, regeneration, and stem cell therapy. It is somewhat controversial, but it is a type of treatment that has received wide publicity due to its usage by famous sports stars who get injured, and who want to heal fast to be in competitive sports.

The patient's blood is drawn and then centrifuged to prepare a concentrated sediment part that is rich in platelets, growth factors, and protein molecules. This is injected into the injured area along with a local anesthetic. It is reported to be useful for faster healing of tennis elbow, tendinitis, and ligament injuries. The exact mechanism of how it works is still not clear. Probably it helps to reduce intra-muscular bleeding by the clotting factors in it and to help it heal faster due to growth factors in it.

Insurance companies do not approve of the treatment since it has not been scientifically researched to have benefits. However it shows the power of our cells, and our body to be able to muster up and heal or regenerate. Some commercial firms publicize this as stem cell treatment.

Regeneration: A feature of living organisms is the capacity to regenerate. Regeneration is the restoration of tissues or organs after injury. Certain reptiles can regrow nearly half of their body even if cut into half. The human body can regrow and heal to some extent. Normal healing of wounds and ulcers are well known. Half of a liver can be removed and the rest of the liver can regrow to a full size. Certain organs can be partially or completely removed with no side effects. We can take out the appendix, gall bladder, spleen, tonsils, and part of the large intestine with very little side effects. Cells from the skin and other tissues can be grown to larger size tissues outside the body by culture techniques. Cells from the body including sperms and ovum can be stored deep-frozen for years to be used at a later date and even create a new baby by in vitro fertilization.

An open wound goes through certain steps to heal itself. Initially, there is a stage of inflammation. At this phase there is swelling due to fluid leak from the blood vessels, allowing white blood cells to come to the area to reduce the infection, the platelets to come in to reduce bleeding. The immune system gets activated. Subsequently, there is a proliferative phase during which repair starts with the migration of fibroblasts, angiogenesis, fibroplasia, and epithelialization. Finally, there is a maturation phase when the scar tightens, and the tissue remodels. The study of wound healing is a subject by itself. The body knows about the injury and tries its best to heal itself, and as soon as it happens.

Continued development of technology is making its mark to aid regeneration and healing of wounds. Molecular biology and tissue engineering are new fields in medicine. It is possible to regrow one's non-functioning organs in the future, making further progress towards the goal of immortality.

Growth And Development: One certainty of life is to have changes in the organism continuously. From the single cell at inception, it grew into a full-blown human body in just 9 months. The changes go on and on and never stop until life ends in the form of death.

A newborn baby shows two features namely growth and development. An increase in size, height, and weight and progress in the behavior, intellect, and social interaction. These changes become evident from infancy and are celebrated as milestones by the parents and family. From the teething to walking, from talking to smiling, from playing to learning, and from crying to hugging, these are cherished memories. The growth goes through childhood to adolescence and finally to adulthood. Women grow and develop faster, but men continue to do so for many more years. Menarche is a marker of adulthood for women while men take another 4 or 5 years to reach a comparable stage. Another milestone is menopause for females, but men take another 5 or 10 years to reach a comparable stage.

For whatever reason, due to the codes in the DNA, the cells stop differentiating into other tissue cells, but will only grow into the same type of cells after a certain period. And then, that type of growth also stops after a certain number of years. For example, during fetal development, the cells could make any type of organs from the liver to the brain to bone or muscle. After the baby is born, it grows each organ steadily until adulthood. The bones grow in height, muscles develop, and genitalia becomes fully functional, and so forth. Then afterward all the growth stops, but the body only replaces lost cells until an older age. Thereafter, this also stops, and cells get depleted and organs weaken. What makes it grow and what makes it stop?

In addition to the genetic factors, hormones such as growth hormone, nutrition, and environmental factors can affect the growth of the person. Exercise can selectively improve the strength and volume of certain parts of the body. Growth and development are expected norms during the tender age. By the same token aging and death are expected in the older age.

Chapter-29

ADOLESCENCE and ADULTHOOD

Adolescence is a period when a child grows up to be an adult. This is a period of rapid growth and gender identification, which leads to varying degrees of turbulence, confusion, maturation, and emotional changes as well as the development of a stable foundation. Changes are often referred to as pubertal, and the period is called puberty. This period can vary for many years until the person matures.

This is also a period of rapid growth. Initially, it is growth in height and weight. What makes them grow and what codes are contained in the DNA? Compared to the initial zygote that could make any type of organs, now the cells in bone, muscles, and tissues keep multiplying their own type of cells, aided by hormones such as growth hormone and sex hormones. The person can become taller, stronger, and heavier. The osteoclasts in the epiphysis of bones make new bone segments to increase height.

The brain also undergoes further development during this period, particularly concerning cognitive functions and behavioral changes. Neurotransmitter hormones of dopamine, serotonin, and glutamine start influencing the emotions of excitement, socialization, pleasure, mood, and behavior.

Physical activity and avoidance of obesity are critical in adolescent life. Statistics show that obesity among adolescents has increased from 5% in 1980 to 18% now (National Health

Examination Survey). This is directly related to time spent on social media, the Internet, television, and digital games, reducing time spent on physical activities. Socio-economic factors also play a role, with poor people and minorities spending less time on sporting activities.

Pubertal changes occur as the most noticeable event during adolescence. Boys notice facial hair, pubic hair, deepening of the voice, and body mass increase. Genital growth and nocturnal ejaculations occur. Females notice the development of breasts, development of pubic hair, growth of hair, and menstrual changes.

Initially, boys and girls want to be mingling within their gender only and develop friendship and bonding. Later on, this preference changes to be with the members of the opposite sex. Much of the initial sexual encounters are out of curiosity and experimentation. Sometimes this may end up even in unintended pregnancies. They start noticing physical changes in their body and want to compare and contrast with other members of society. They want to declare independence, but they have their shortcomings and inability to do so. Their financial and social dependence on the parents is resented and appreciated at the same time.

The female sex has a clearly defined episode in their life in the form of menarche. It is a statement that the woman has become an adult physiologically. However, she is not mature enough physically or socially to be independent. Men do not have such well-defined events in their life as they take another 4 to 5 years to reach their level of maturity. Their changes are slow and subtle.

This period has the potential for emotional instability if there is not enough understanding and support from parents, families, and friends. They can easily blame their parents for anything that goes wrong. Depression and suicidal tendencies creep in. There is rebellion internally and externally. Parents are at times seen as enemies, and friends at the same time. Unless they are seen as supportive, they have a desire to run away from home, but then they do not know where to go and how to do it. So they feel trapped and shut the doors of their rooms and listen to music or watch television. Parents are seen as old fashioned, possessive, and dictatorial. Friends are seen as pacifiers and peacemakers, and understanding people.

This fragile and volatile period can be made tolerable by the conscious efforts of parents. Adolescents want to be treated as adults and not as children. They want to be consulted instead of being told to do so. Graded responsibilities must be assigned to them to conduct their affairs. Gentle guidance as to the future and need for a solid foundation in the form of education needs to be instilled. Moral values of honesty, integrity, and work ethics have to be demonstrated by the parents. They do not want to be compared with others. They do not want to be put down. They want to be encouraged and appreciated for their achievements, grades, and scores.

Broken families and divorced parents face even more difficulties. Either the mother figure or father figure is missing in their life. They look for help and guidance, but it is missing. Drug addiction and alcoholism of parents automatically transfers to children. A child subjected to abuse, violence, or neglect tends to become derelicts of society.

Adulthood is when growth and development have matured. People make statements such as "grow up" or "behave like an adult" to describe better behavior. Legally it could be 18 or 21 according to rules and regulations. One is considered to have become a major at 18 and can start driving a car and sign for oneself. One can vote for election at 18. The drinking age is 21 in many states.

However, age alone does not make one an adult. Adulthood is also social development. Physical development is one factor. Legal responsibility for one's actions is another factor. It is also how people view each other and more importantly how they view themselves. Many individuals who are 21 or 22 are still in college, very much dependent on their parents, and do not recognize themselves as adults.

Adulthood comes when one has accepted oneself as an adult. Two things matter at this time of life- first is to declare independence with a job and income, and second is to have a relationship with the opposite sex.

Education can continue as an ongoing process, but earning money to live on one's terms becomes a priority. No more handouts from parents, no more feeling of slavery, no more begging. It feels good to be independent and self-supportive. A job brings self-esteem more than anything else in life. It is not just the money, not just the income. It is the feeling that you are worthy of somebody. You are doing something meaningful. You are contributing to society, and you are supporting your family. However, for many individual's education involves a college degree and additional professional qualifications, postponing job hunting until the age of 25 to 30.

Sex is a natural phenomenon intended for progeny and the creation of future generations. For the purpose of fertilization, to create the new zygote, it is necessary to bring the ovum and sperm into contact. Without such an urge and a pleasurable experience, there would be no procreation. Genitals were intentionally created by nature as sensitive and exhilarating organs so that natural interest in having sex would occur. It is the society where we live in, that has made restrictions in the form of customs, rules, and regulations. Societal norms expect one to be in a marriage to have sex and children. This leads to certain amounts of stress, depression, and violence, since many couples do not get along. Left to the law of nature, people would have sex more freely.

Genetically and biologically men are prone to be polygamous and women are more often monogamous. One could see this phenomenon in the animal kingdom also. Male species want to spread their sperms as quickly as possible with as many female species as possible, whereas the female species are more interested in being a homemaker, child-bearer, and want to be in a safe and secure environment.

In her book, "*Not always in the mood: The new science of Men, sex and relationships*" Sarah Hunter Murray describes that men are branded as being dark, selfish, and abusive, without understanding them. The "Me too Movement" is interested in putting down the entire male species as rapists, molesters, and harassers. Believing that men are interested in only one thing, to have sex all the time. This is far from the truth. Men are looking for emotional support and bonding more often, and their emotions and needs are not well appreciated. They want to feel needed and comforted. Sarah Hunter Murray has done extensive interviews and research on this topic for over 10 years. What drives a man is the feeling of being connected and being close, much more than the physical attraction. Without intimacy and being on the same page, sex becomes dull and less enjoyable.

A midlife crisis sets in for both men and women. Again, for women, there is a clearly defined biological event in the form of menopause. No more ova are made every month. No more childbearing. Nature has decided no further reproductive use for the woman. There could be emotional, behavioral, and physical changes in the postmenopausal period. PMS (Postmenopausal stress) is a real entity. Manifestations may begin in the form of flushing, sweating, emotional outbursts, and mood swings. Hormonal changes may lead to osteoporosis, cancers, and heart attacks.

Men do not have a well-defined biological event similar to menopause in women. However, they do undergo periods of depression, emotional disturbances, feeling of having wasted their life, and worthlessness in midlife. They see life as slipping away. Obesity, alcoholism, and drug addiction creeps in. Job security is not a guarantee and the fear of being fired and replaced by a younger person is real. Divorces, suicides, and bankruptcies occur. More pressure and stress exist on men than on women and it manifests as heart attacks and strokes.

A focused and determined effort must be made during adulthood to maintain good physical and mental health. One should plan for good retirement with financial security and good health. That means avoiding alcohol and drug addictions, maintaining proper body weight by watching the diet, and exercising adequately. Adequate sleep and rest are needed and must be worked into the daily schedule. Family and friends are important and one's social life reduces tension and stress. A willful effort has to be made to socialize and to find hobbies.

SECTION- 8 - Prevention of death

Chapter 30

PREVENTABLE CAUSES OF DEATH

Improving life expectancy equates with prolonging life or postponing death. It is a path seeking immortality. Already we are living double the number of years compared to those who were born 200 years ago. It is possible we can still double it in the next 100 years if we pay attention to causes that bring in premature death.

Various recommendations and advice on maintenance of good health, by doctors and insurance companies, and other health care advocates, are ignored by a large number of people.

Over 50% of illnesses and over 50% of the hospitalizations are due to lifestyle issues. Just take the following few situations that account for most such calamities:

- Smoking, Heavy drinking, Drug addiction
- Obesity, Stress, and anger
- Loss of family structure, divorces
- Gun violence, Road accidents
- Lack of exercise, Poor medical check-ups
- Preventable medical errors, Suicides
- Ignorance about vaccinations and preventive health care.

To give you an idea, smoking causes 400,000 deaths a year, improper diet causes 300,000 deaths a year and alcohol causes 100,000 deaths a year.

Vaccinations have helped to ward off infectious diseases and related mortality and morbidity to an innumerable number of people, and have helped to prolong a good quality of life for many. Still, there are many people in the United States, let alone underdeveloped countries, who question the value of vaccinations and avoid taking them for fear of unsubstantiated allegations. Thousands of people used to die from smallpox, chickenpox, measles, polio, and diphtheria, and tetanus. Malaria and plague have been controlled with the understanding of the role of vectors such as mosquitoes and rats. Salmonella, Shigella, HIV/ AIDS, and many other insect born infections and parasitic infestations have been controlled with good health habits, sanitation precautions, hand washing, and proper cooking of food and water. Still, thousands die every year because of ignorance, poverty, abuse, and negligence.

Despite these various causes of death, and danger lingering everywhere, it must be recognized that people live almost double the life span now compared to 200 years ago. Life expectancy in 1900 for all sexes was 47.3 years. In 2015 it was 78.8 years, according to a WHO study. It was very common for children to die at a young age, mothers to die from childbirth, many young people to die from communicable diseases, and natural disasters and wars. Science has made progress by leaps and bounds. We have a better understanding of anesthesia, asepsis, surgery, we have many wonder drugs, and we have controlled many parasitic and communicable diseases. We have postponed death to a much later date.

Chapter 31

HOMICIDES

Mass shootings from gun violence are common in the United States of America. Nearly 50 people die every day from gun violence alone; nearly 40,000 people die needlessly every year. The National Rifle Association and the gun lobby have a stronghold on the politicians. They hang on to the second amendment of the constitution as the excuse. They want to keep a gun in their house to protect themselves from intruders and to use them for hunting, entertainment, and sporting. Many mass shootings are common such as the Parkland High School shooting in Florida, the Las Vegas shooting, the Orlando night club shooting, the Newport Elementary School shooting in Connecticut, and the Santa Fe School shooting in Texas. After each shooting, the community gathers for prayer and candlelight vigils, the politicians give the same speech expressing their condolences; the media have a hay day of news and coverage. After about a week or two, they go back to life as usual until the next event occurs. It has been proven beyond doubt that the countries that have gun control laws have low gun-related deaths. However, this is a faraway dream in the United States, because everyone loves his or her guns.

Newspaper reports in September of 2018 showed a marked increase in killings in Latin America last year. 400 murders were reported to be happening every day in just four countries together- Brazil, Venezuela, Mexico, and Colombia. With only 8% of the world population, Latin America was accounting for one-third of global murders. One out of four of all murders in the world was taking place in these countries alone. In one city of Acapulco, which used to be a tourist haven, the deaths have erased that image. With a population of 800,000, there were 953 murders in one year alone, more killings than Italy, Spain, Switzerland, Portugal, and the Netherlands put together. El Salvador's murder rate of 83 per 100,000 people in 2016 was the highest rate of murders in any country, which was nearly 17 times that of the US.

People have become so used to the murders, to the extent that they keep eating food in the cafeteria while killings are going on right in front of their shop. Refugees flee the countries in large numbers to escape gangs like MS13 and Barrio 18. Bodies pile up in the morgue before they can be processed. Trucks carrying the corpses were roaming for two and three days, looking to dump them in a morgue. Up to 10% of the cadavers are never claimed. No one bothers to file a police report or pick up a body. Sometimes only body parts such as a limb or torsos are dumped.

Latin America accounts for 43 of the 50 most murderous countries. All of the top 10 such cities are located in Latin America. If you live in one of these cities, there is a 1 in 10 chance that you will get murdered over eventually. Between 2000 and 2017, 2.5 million people have been thus killed in Latin America and the Caribbean combined. This compares with a total of 900,000 killed in armed conflicts of Syria, Iraq, and Afghanistan combined.

Murder tallies may be under-reported since many deaths are untraceable. The victims are tossed into unmarked graves, or dissolved with acid. There are hundreds and thousands of bone fragments belonging to unidentified victims. More than 62 million have fled their homes or countries.

One of the main causes of this state is poverty and a history of violence in the system. Bloody wars were needed for the independence of new governments. The widest gap between rich and poor is noted here, fueling resentment. Corruption, illegal trades, family-owned business unaccountable to the government, the culture of drug cartels, power groups running local affairs are all factors. Rapid urbanization without infrastructure, schools, and hospitals are increasing the number of single-parent homes, and lawlessness has created vicious cycles.

Organized crime flourishes here with mafia-type lords due to coco plants being grown and converted to cocaine drugs, ready to be exported to a high demand country in the neighborhood, which is the US. There are also many family quarrels, which end up being violent following drinking parties.

In the 1950s, Singapore and Caracas had similar high violence rates. After independence in 1962, the authoritarian regimen under Lew Kwan Yew established strict laws, boosted education, work ethics, and social integration. Now it has a very low violence rate. Wherever there is a weak legal system and police system, people take the law into their own hands and kill for trivial reasons.

Murder by definition is depriving another person of life against their will. However, all such deaths are not considered murder by society. Mass murders routinely take place in times of war, by the justification that it is a premeditated decision of you against me. The so-called 'Stand the ground' is a legally permitted killing in most states, stating that it was done for self-defense. Ethnic cleansing and riots are often initiated and instigated by the politicians in power. Mercy killings or euthanasia and physician-assisted suicides take place due to underlying medical problems. Killings were authorized by the society from time to time because of blasphemy, an accusation of corrupting the minds of youth, going against local customs, interracial weddings, sexual orientations, and adultery and prostitution. Such "honor killings" are well known in Pakistan, Afghanistan, and several other Islamic countries, to enforce their moral values in their societies. Capital punishment is an intentional killing by the government to invoke fear in the public mind to maintain law and order.

There are more guns in the US than the population of the country. According to a survey in 2015, it was noted that 22%

of people own guns. Each person has an average of 4.8 guns. Gun violence is a preventable disease. Solutions must be found to reduce this catastrophe.

The habit of owning guns go back to the origin of the nation. Independence was won with a war against England, in which many ordinary citizens participated. Also, the civil war. The Second Amendment of the Constitution guaranteed "the right to keep and bear arms" with a "well-regulated militia". At that time much of America was rural, and a gun was needed for protection and hunting. It was a tool for most families, sporting equipment, and was a family tradition. Yet times have changed, most people live in cities or suburbs. Few go hunting to get food and there are rules and regulations along with law and order in the society. Homes with guns have more shootings and deaths compared to homes without guns. Accidental shootings, suicidal as well as homicidal shootings occur because of the availability of the gun.

Most of the killings with guns are suicides- about two-thirds of them. School shootings have become more common, to the extent that teachers are asked to carry guns to protect them and metal detectors are installed at school entrances.

New Zealand was a generally peaceful country, but a mass killing occurred in March 2019, by a racially motivated murderer killing over 40 people in a mosque. The Government immediately announced strict gun control laws, unlike the US. Unfortunately, the ISIS and Moslem groups decided to take revenge. They conducted a terrorist attack in Sri Lanka, with suicide bombs and gun violence in a coordinated fashion to kill nearly 300 Christians on the Easter day. Three churches during Easter services and three luxury hotels were targeted. Over 400 people were injured. It is so sad that religious riots and conflicts result in so many mass deaths even with so much education and knowledge and awareness all across the globe.

Chapter 32

PREVENTABLE MEDICAL ERRORS

Preventable medical error is the third leading cause of death in the United States, after heart attacks and cancers. About 200,000 people die from preventable medical errors every year.

With an advanced health care system, marvelous technology, and highly qualified and credentialed doctors and nurses, it would be hard to believe that so many mistakes occur. No one makes an error intentionally. However, the system allows things to fall through the cracks. The patient and family need to be vigilant and avoid unnecessary medical treatments and hospitalizations.

Doctors and nurses and other health care professionals start their careers with the best intentions. They are smart, noble-minded, and hard working. At any given time they want to do the best for their patients. Why do these errors occur then? Part of the answer is that they become immune to the human side of medicine after some time. It becomes just work, and more work to meet the regulations. They have to prioritize their time. Routines are assumed to be the standards after some time so that in the crowded emergency room, the one who comes by ambulance, or the one brought in by cops get to be seen first. Someone with a headache or vomiting gets pushed into a corner waiting for four or six hours, even if they may be having a serious condition. Many items are missed between changes of hands, change of shifts, and are lost in the shuffle. A test result or a report may get more attention than a physical examination or history taking.

Patient's names are forgotten and at times they are addressed as "patient in bed no 2 or the case in isolation or the one in the corner room' or refer to them as the working diagnosis as 'the gall bladder in bed no 3' or the asthma case in the 4th cubicle. The cases all run together and feel the same. The doctors are focused on getting their work done rather than treating the patient as a person. They learn to detach from personal involvement so that they can cope up with the stress of the work. The advice is don't get emotional and don't get too close.

Those who experience bad outcomes are more likely to be poor than rich and more likely to be black than white and more likely to be uninsured than insured. This is because underprivileged people do not seek medical attention early on, often go to the emergency room instead of private doctors, are uninformed about health care needs, and afraid of the doctors and medical system in general.

In the United States, many new technological and unproven treatments are often adopted with the label of being the most advanced or the latest. Some of these procedures, technical achievements, or treatment modalities turn out to be unhelpful, unnecessary, and often harmful to the patient. Many people die in the process or acquire severe complications. These incidents are written off as part of the process. However, during the introduction period, these modalities of treatment are widely publicized by the hospital and doctors as marketing tools. Truly speaking it is the drug companies and equipment manufacturers who are the big beneficiaries.

Lasers were the hype at one time for all abdominal surgery for doing minimally invasive surgery. It took some time to recognize that laparoscopy helps and not lasers. In the process, millions of dollars were spent on lasers and hundreds of patients died from lasers. Now it has gone on to the hype of using robotics for everything that can be done with a simple incision and suture. A hernia repair can be done with no special equipment; then it became a laparoscopic procedure, and now it is a robotic procedure. The cost has become 1,000 times more compared to the old-fashioned incision procedure. There is no difference in the outcome and there are more complications, but this is the fashion of the day. If a surgeon does not use robotics, that surgeon becomes old fashioned and outdated. The practice of medicine has become competitive for money and fame.

Repair of a hiatal hernia by surgery was very popular at one time, now it is way down. Placement of a gastric band for weight reduction was very popular- now it is abandoned. The Federal government recently banned the use of meshes for vaginal prolapse after numerous complications.

Stem cell therapy and high dose chemotherapy was a treatment for all metastatic cancers, only to be found that many patients died and most had severe complications, and there was no improvement. Each time the stem cell chemotherapy or otherwise commonly known as bone marrow transplantation was used the total bill came to almost one million dollars. Insurance companies refused to cover it as unproven, but patients sued the insurance companies. The final result was that it did not work, and the whole process has been abandoned. Many innocent people died, and millions of dollars were charged by the health care system. No single person is to be blamed, but it was the culture, it was the right thing to do at that time, and everyone believed in it. Between 1989 and 2001, about 40,000 people received this type of treatment, only to be found that it did not make any difference in their outcome afterward.

Similarly, many drugs come and go, many operations come and go, many instruments come and go. However, many people suffer during the time.

Another problem is an excessive number of tests are done much more than are necessary. This not only increases the cost but also causes harm. The patient receives an ultrasound, then a CT scan, followed by an MRI scan and then a PET scan, followed by some other invasive tests. There is an acronym in a surgery called VOMIT, which stands for victims of modern imaging technology. A questionable something is seen in one of the tests, which leads to more tests, and then an invasive procedure for further diagnosis or treatment. Then it leads to complications and more surgery, which snowballs into more medical problems. Moreover, excessive radiation from x-rays can cause cancers. It is estimated that 1% of cancers in the US are caused by excessive radiation from medical imaging. We have seen CT scans being repeated every other day several times to follow the progress of severely ill patients.

We tend to accept that anything introduced new should be good, any new technology must be better, and anything that gets advertised or written up in the media must be tried. We forget the time-tested methods of clinical diagnosis and treatment.

Chapter 33

SUICIDES

"Happiness in intelligent people is the rarest thing I know"-
wrote Ernest Hemingway, who committed suicide by gunshot
in 1961.

About 50,000 people committed suicide last year in the US.
The Center for Disease Control calls it a disease that can be
prevented. All across the world, 2000 people commit suicide
daily and twice the number attempt it unsuccessfully. They felt
that their lives were unworthy. They were disenchanted with
life. What made them think so?

Sometimes it is a depression or a mental disorder,
sometimes it is a feeling of failure in life. Sometimes they feel
that suicide is the right thing to do. Within the United States,
Utah ranks highest in depression and suicides. Montana and
New Mexico and other mountain states follow. It could be the
isolation, weather conditions, dusky landscape that contribute
to mental depression. There is an uptick in the number of
suicides during Springtime and to a lesser extent during Fall,
unlike the common perception that cold winter months may
cause brooding. The precise cause of the spring peak in
suicides is unclear. Possible theories include longer days with
light, allergy to pollens, and changes in the immune system.

In the US, suicide is the 10th leading cause of death in all
ages, but for young people, it is the second most common cause
of death, after accidents. In the year 2017, there were 47,126
deaths from suicide and nearly 1.4 million attempted suicides
were recorded. While males commit more suicides, females

make more attempts to commit suicide. Prior mental health problems and prior attempts at suicides are forewarning signs. The cost of medical care and work loss costs are estimated to be $70 billion per year from suicides and attempted suicides.

Cults and clans can persuade one to suicide. One of the largest mass suicides in history was in Jonestown, Guyana, when 918 people committed mass suicide, by drinking a poisoned cool drink at the calling of Rev. Jim Jones, the head of the cult on Nov 18, 1978. There were some murders also associated with the event. The town was built in the jungle of Guyana, South America at the behest of Jim Jones as a cult community.

People decide to commit suicide when they have reached a breaking point in their lives. They do not want to live anymore due to massive depression and hopelessness. They feel there is no meaningful purpose to live and earn. They see only a dark ally in front of them. Everything they hoped for is snubbed out. There is no more option, no more choice, no more objectives, no more anguish or suffering. Their decision is at times due to actions by their family members, at times due to their illnesses, or mental disorder, or financial losses. Highly successful men who get involved deeply in their work can forget to live a balanced life, and suddenly they find themselves in a dark hole. Many actors like Marilyn Monroe, singers like Michael Jackson, business people like Kate Spades, Television celebrities like Antony Bourdain committed suicide. Surgeons are one group of professionals with a high rate of divorces, suicides, and bankruptcies, caused by stress and total dedication to their work.

I like to recite the story of two of my physician friends who committed suicide in the prime of their lives. The first one was a tall and handsome Caucasian of Australian descent, a smart and polite surgeon who went to an Ivy League college and medical school in the US, started a very successful practice in my town, and had a very busy practice. He was in the operating room or hospital most of the time and his wife divorced him due to poor family life. He fell for a scrub nurse who trapped him. He married her and continued with his busy practice. After a year or so, she started an affair with another person since he was never home. He felt dejected and worthless in life and took his own life.

The other was a successful plastic surgeon again very busy and dedicated. He put all the money he earned in his wife's name for fear of the potential for medical malpractice claims. One day the wife left him with all the money for another man. He pulled the trigger at his head sitting in his office room.

Why do people commit suicide? Is it possible that there is an innate desire for everyone to die on our own accord and we are suppressing it with our cerebral thinking? Do the animals show a desire for suicide? We would think that survival is their innate attitude. Is it the depression that sets in or is it a drug addiction? Depression is four times more common among women than men, but men are twice as likely to commit suicide from depression than women. Single people are more likely to commit suicide than married people. Religious minds are less likely to kill themselves, leaving the burden to God. Those who commit suicide have been mulling over it for a long time, they have been thinking about it at least for a while. They may act on a spur of the moment, but the thought process is entertained for some time. There is a feeling of being a burden to others, and the perception of being unwanted or not belonging here. There is a feeling of emptiness, a feeling that no one cares. Divorced men commit suicide 400 times more than divorced women. Nearly half of those committing suicide have seen a doctor or talked to a friend within a month or two before the final act. Sometimes they have talked about it or given warning signs to others in subtle ways. If you are a male above the age of sixty-five, divorced and in poor health, living alone in a metropolitan area, having a gun in your house, you are at high risk for committing suicide. Men more often shoot themselves with a gun, while women more often use poison or make self-inflicted wounds. Dark, cold winter months make them brood, but actual suicides are more common in spring. Most of them leave a note explaining their action, saying goodbye, and making clear their motives. Some of the notes are brief while others are voluminous. Some people now tape record or video record their final message.

The views about suicides have changed from time to time. Ancient Greeks and Romans felt it was a noble thing to do since their punishment for breaking the law or losing a war could be more humiliating and torturous. By the 6th century, suicide was considered a sin, and then an attempted suicide was considered an offense or crime.

Further later in the nineteenth-century literature and poetry began to portray it as an act of romance. Many love stories were written where the lovers found suicide was the final act of their union. The story of Cleopatra and Mark Anthony goes back two thousand years ago. A fake note of suicide by Cleopatra, as a conspiracy to get him out of power, was given to Mark Anthony. Deeply in love with her, he then committed suicide on his sword. Hearing this the Cleopatra had a poisonous snake bite her intentionally to volunteer her death. They were buried together. Shakespeare wrote the story of Romeo and Juliet. Many melodrama movies have been made with lovers committing suicide together, to fight against injustice by the families or societies.

Subsequent years show it as an act of self-control, to be able to decide one's fate by themselves rather than by destiny at an unknown time and unknown way. If suicide can be considered to have a genetic predisposition, Ernest Hemingway's suicide at age 67 is an example. His father shot himself at age of 57, two of his siblings also took their own lives, and his son and granddaughter also did the same.

Research shows that Dialectical Behavior Therapy (DBT) can be an effective tool to help people with suicidal ideations. Careful observation and follow-up of those with depression are needed. They should be prevented from owning guns or such tools for suicide since many suicides are impulsively committed. They may have talked about suicide, and even had attempted it in the past. Talking to them gently and with compassion will help to delay such action. DBT teaches patients how to manage their emotions, how to have stronger relationships and communications. It teaches them how to cope up with stressful situations, and crisis management. It encourages them to exercise, socialize, eat well, and sleep well. Depression is treated with medications early on. A national suicide prevention lifeline can also provide resources. The hotline for the same is 800-273-8255

Suicides were considered acceptable and at times an honorable thing to do from pre-historic times. In Japan, it was known as Hari-kari. When the king or soldiers were defeated, they would rather commit suicide in the field than getting captured as prisoners and be tortured. They did not want to become slaves, and women folk did not want to become mistresses. In ancient Greek culture, suicide was allowed under certain circumstances in society, and could even request the government for help. Suicide was a form of punishment too. The famous philosopher Socrates was asked to drink hemlock poison in 399 B.C. as a court-ordered punishment for attempting to corrupt the minds of youngsters.

In India, during the Muslim rule, the practice of Sati started. When the husband died the wife was expected to self-immolate herself in the funeral pyre of the husband. The practice is illegal and banned now. At that time there was a real fear of a widow being subjected to sexual and other abuses. When a kingdom was defeated in war, many women committed mass suicides in large fire pits for the same reason. Another news report from India revealed that over 300,000 farmers have committed suicide in the last 10-year period due to financial struggles, draught, and corrupt practices.

Suicides are increasing in numbers in the United States. More middle-aged people are committing suicides than before. It is estimated that 45,000 people commit suicides every year in the US. A new statistics issued by the CDC in August of 2018 shows that 72,000 people committed suicide due to opioid drug abuse alone. About 750 a year kill their loved ones and then commit suicide for medical reasons. They just cannot stand the prolonged agony and suffering of loved ones. This may be an act of compassion or an act of desperation for escape. Over 50% of the suicides in the US are by using guns.

In an article published in the Journal of American College of Surgeons in August 2018, exact statistics issued by the Center for Disease Control and Prevention for the year 2016 is quoted. There were 63,979 intentional injury deaths, making it an average of 175 deaths every single day. Out of these 44,867, (70%) of deaths were suicides and 19103 (30%) were homicides. Out of the suicides, the cause of death was gunshot wounds self-inflicted in 22,938 (51%). Out of the homicides, 14,415 (75%) involved the use of firearms. This works out to be 37,353 deaths total (58%) with the use of firearms. Since 1999, there is a 17% increase in the use of firearms for all intentional injury deaths and a 20% increase by all mechanisms of intentional injury deaths in the US. In the same period, deaths from traffic-related accidents decreased by 22%.

If you are having a suicidal tendency or thought, call the National Suicide Prevention Lifeline at 1-800-273-8255 (TALK) or go to Speaking of Suicide.com/resources, or suicidepreventionlifeline.org

Suicide or attempted suicide by a person is not illegal in any of the States in the US. While suicide itself is not a crime, a botched suicide, an unsuccessful one where someone assisted to commit suicide, or where someone caused enough emotional trauma to make the person commit suicide, or where someone encouraged the person to commit suicide can all get prosecuted as a crime. There have been so many stories about such incidents. In the dorm of a college, someone took a video of another student with a homosexual act and put it on social media, which resulted in that individual committing suicide. The offender was penalized. There was another incident where one female student motivated another one to commit suicide, which resulted in her legal trouble. Hazing in college dorms, constant bullying, discrimination, and isolation have been causes of suicide and they are treated as crimes against those individuals.

One well-known story of a botched physician-assisted suicide was the trial of Dr. Peter Rosier in 1988 in Florida. His wife was suffering from terminal cancer, and she wanted to end her life with help of her family. After a family reunion and bidding farewell, she went to bed and took twenty pills of seconal, a barbiturate, which had been obtained with help of her husband. She went into a deep coma but was still alive in the morning. Her husband then gave her morphine, but still, she was breathing after several hours. At that point, he went into her room and suffocated her with no resistance what so ever. After the period of mourning and cremation, things would have been quiet except the husband made a big mistake when he wrote a book about her and also went on live television telling how he had helped to end her life. The State's attorney general initiated a lawsuit against the husband and family. The jury acquitted the husband after a lengthy trial. There have been several instances where a lawsuit had been filed against physician-assisted suicide over terminally ill patients. However, all of them have been acquitted.

Murder and suicides are both forms of killing. Yet we generally tend to see them differently. We feel outraged with a murderer and want to have the person punished, often with capital punishment or outright killing of the murderer in revenge. Whereas we feel sorry for the person who committed suicide.

According to an article published in the Wall Street Journal on Nov.29, 2018 by Betsy McKay, CDC (Center for Disease Control) reported that suicides are increasing in the United States to the extent that life expectancy was reduced in this country last year. Now the life expectancy in the US is 78.9 years compared to 84.1 years in Japan and 83.7 years in Switzerland. A good number of suicides are related to opioid addiction. The CDC (Center for Disease Control) also reported that there were a total of 2.8 million deaths in the US last year, up 70,000 more deaths compared to the previous year. The breakdown reveals that deaths from cancers came down, but deaths from suicides especially related to opioid addiction and gun violence went up. Deaths from cardiac causes remained unchanged. Deaths from suicides are 14 per 100,000people, the highest since 1975.

Chapter 34

ENVIRONMENTAL PROBLEMS AND POLLUTION

Air pollution in New Delhi is so high that living there one day is equal to smoking 50 cigarettes that one day. The rating of pollution in New Delhi recently was 1000, as compared to 35 to 40 in most of the US. Seven million people die from the after-effects of air pollution each year. Much of the air pollution is man-made. Carbon emissions from cars and factories can be reduced to help the cause. Air pollution is different from global warming and climate change.

Climate change is real. More people are dying recently due to extreme weather conditions. We experience more heatwaves with resultant wildfires, more cold climates in other parts of the world, hurricanes, tornados, tsunamis, floods, and rains all across the globe. Excessive heat and cold weathers are harmful, resulting in the deaths of hundreds of people every year. Polar ice is melting and glaciers are melting in front of our eyes. There is a dispute as to the cause of global warming. Some think it is due to carbon emission and loss of the greenhouse effect from the reduced ozone layer. Others think it is due to planet alignments that change periodically.

Environmental pollution can occur in different forms. Chemical discharges from factories seep into groundwater or open waters and can cause damage to fish and animals as well as poison people. Fracking for shale oil production requires water under high pressure to be pumped deep underground which causes contamination of the soil and underground waters. Industrial pollution is evident in open waters, groundwaters, or the atmosphere.

Contamination of the Ganges River with discharges of wastes, human excreta, and dead bodies is notorious. Untreated sewage is discharged into the rivers that teem with bacteria. Devotees want to take a dip in the river for washing off their sins and to stop the cycle of reincarnations, but they suffer from the effects of the polluted river and contagious illnesses.

Noise can also be a pollutant. Too much noise and smells are harmful. Religious organizations compete to blast their prayers at all odd hours, waking up people from sleep intermittently. Garbage disposal is a health hazard in many undeveloped countries. Everyone just throws the garbage including plastic bottles and plastic bags out on the road and the beaches and waterways. They are not biodegradable, they cause a smell, rot, and decay, encouraging certain larvae, rats, and animals to grow in these areas, plug up drainage pipes and waterways causing illnesses to humans.

Lack of sanitation facilities forces people to urinate and defecate in open spaces. These cause contamination of plants and vegetables, encourage rape and sexual crimes, and enable parasitic infestations. Wandering animals such as stray dogs, cows, goats and buffaloes, monkeys, and birds cause contaminations and transmission of animal bite-related diseases.

Radioactive pollution and contamination occur from time to time due to nuclear plants having defective issues. The Chernobyl incident is an example. There have been nuclear power plant leakage incidents in the US such as the Love Canal incident. The whole region becomes uninhabitable, people get various illnesses and cancers and result in many deaths. The adverse effects can linger for many years. The proliferation of nuclear weapons by different countries for power and control has no end in sight. Disposal of radioactive waste products from these establishments is a real problem.

Lead paints, radon, and molds inside houses can create health issues. Toys contaminated with lead have led to neurological deficits in children. Contaminated food, fruits, and strawberries from the fields have caused salmonella, cholera, and E. Coli infections. The excess lead was noted in the water supply in Flint, Michigan. Excess groundwater fluoride is seen in Bihar, India that causes severe skeletal damages.

Chapter 35

ACCIDENTS

Road accidents kill scores of people all over the globe. Pedestrian deaths from automobiles hitting them have increased to a 30-year high number of 6227 in 2018 according to the national highway safety association in the US. The distraction of drivers with cellphones, lack of adequate protection for pedestrians, high-speed driving, and lack of adequate lighting are felt as factors. Pedestrians also share some of the responsibilities.

Drowning is the third most common cause of accidental deaths in the US, after road accidents and violence. Nearly half a million people die from drowning worldwide every year. While most people die in open waters such as lakes, rivers, and seas and from natural disasters of floods, paradoxically in the United States and Australia most victims drown in swimming pools.

The average person can hold their breath for a maximum of one and a half minutes. The brain suffers permanent damage after four minutes without oxygen. During drowning, the air passages become filled with water during the effort to breathe underwater and the person dies of choking. However, under cold water people can survive up to 10 minutes after drowning because of the effects of hypothermia.

Plane accidents have become lesser in numbers with increased air safety regulations and computerization. Yet each airplane accident causes major media publicity due to the shocking number of people dying at one instance suddenly.

Some of the worst plane accidents have remained unresolved. More recently two of the plane crashes were related to aircraft defects in Boeing 787 Max 8 system.

Accidents occur at various workplaces and factories and construction sites. Injury-related to the use of machinery, equipment, construction can result in permanent disability or death. The mining industry has had instances of accidents, and health care problems such as the black lung.

The defense department sends soldiers to protect and defend the country. Many can get killed or disabled in the line of duty. Fireworks related to festival times or holidays can result in blast injuries and burns. Fire in workplace areas and buildings are due to electrical shorts or other code violations.

Many of the accidents and related deaths are preventable. Safety precautions while driving, wearing seat belts, avoiding distractions, avoiding the use of cell phones while driving, avoiding driving while tired, under the influence of alcohol or drugs, or driving when sleepy are common-sense measures that will significantly reduce accidents. Keeping toddlers indoors, making sure they do not get to the swimming pools without supervision, teaching them swimming lessons to save themselves, and avoiding jumping from heights into the waters are helpful to minimize drowning incidents. Workplace safety, hazard recognition, factory regulations, availability of health care support, and proper human resource management are measures to reduce industrial accidents.

Accidents take another 40,000 lives each year. Automobile accidents that happen on the road take the vast share. Some of the accidents are destiny and happens for no one's fault. However, some of the accidents are due to negligence, carelessness, and ignorance.

Bicycle accidents are common in communities where the road conditions are not good for the cyclers. In certain countries such as Denmark, Sweden, China, and Baltic nations cycling is common and there are good bicycle lanes. However, in the US and many other Asian and African countries, the cycles have to share the same road with motorists, leading to accidents. A Wall Street Journal article on September 26, 2018, gives information on cycle deaths in the US. There were 840 deaths from cycle accidents in the year 2016, which is a 35% increase compared to 2010. The highest number of deaths is in the State of Florida due to several tourists driving on unfamiliar roads, few designated bike lanes, and a tendency for distractions while driving such as texting, alcohol intake, poorly lit county roads, and the older population.

Chapter 36

DRUG ADDICTION

Opioid addiction kills over 70,000 people a year in the US. Much of the new addiction is related to synthetic drugs such as fentanyl that have become available in the market.

Drug addiction has often been traced to the doctor's office as the starting point. About twenty years ago doctors were chastised for prescribing inadequate pain medication. Pain management specialties sprung up. The pendulum swung too far, and now the complaint is that doctors are prescribing too many pain medications and narcotics. Patients demand instant pain relief with narcotics such as Vicodin, Percocet, morphine, Dilaudid, Pethidine, and Oxycontin. Patients wanted refills several times, which led to addictive habits. Moreover, many patients have chronic pain syndromes, fibromyalgia, fatigue syndrome, and chronic back pain and arthritic conditions.

When the government and third-party insurances started clamping down on excess pain management prescriptions, patients went hunting for drugs in the street. Cocaine, heroin, angel dust, methadone, and synthetics such as fentanyl and meth were in high demand. Behavioral problems, family disruptions, emotional issues, and peer pressure and depression further contribute to drug addiction.

Sharing needles, careless personal conduct, and overdose problems lead to HIV/AIDS, infections of various natures, respiratory illnesses, coma, and cardiac arrest. 5% of newborns in America are exposed to opioid drugs in utero. The opioid addiction has become an epidemic, which if left unchecked will kill 500,000 people in the next 7 years.

There have been little efforts so far by the government or politicians to stem the tide. Corporations that make the drugs and the drug lords who share the profit with distributors are unhinged. Deaths that occur at a slow pace, one death at a time does not alarm the society compared to mass shootings. The White House Council of Economic Advisers estimates a total social cost as high as $504billion a year due to the opioid crisis, whereas, a bipartisan bill last year allocated just $1 billion for a two year period to address the issue.

Chapter 37

DO's and DON'Ts to live longer

DO's

Control and watch your diet
Exercise regularly
Control your weight
Reduce your stress
Go for regular medical check-ups
Follow your doctor's advice
You must know your diagnosis, medications, and treatment plans
You have a right to refuse treatment
You have a right to obtain a second opinion
Keep all paperwork, Living Wills, and durable power of attorneys in order
Have friends, family, and a social circle
Get married, have children
Stay engaged with brain activities
Live in a healthy place with minimum pollution
Use safe sex precautions
Wash your hands frequently
Floss your teeth and brush teeth regularly
Use a proper toilet
Bathe or shower daily
Use a skin moisturizer or oil
Use sunscreen lotion
Use sunglasses
Use insect repellents

Use mosquito net
Drive safely
Wear a seat belt in vehicles and airplanes
Wear a helmet while driving any type of two-wheelers
Prayer, peace, and accept destiny or God
Relaxation techniques
Sleep well
Listen to music
Have hobbies
Go to a temple or place of worship
Meditate
Volunteer to help less the fortunate

Covid Precautions

Maintain social distancing of at least 6 feet apart
Wear a mask when in proximity to others
Avoid large gatherings
Avoid unnecessary travels.
Outdoor sporting activities and outdoor seatings are better
Get tested when in doubt.
Self-quarantine after travels or when in contact with infected persons
Wash your hands frequently
Avoid touching your face and nose frequently
Use hand sanitizer as needed
Clean and wipe off surfaces that you touch frequently
Report high fever or flu-like symptoms to your doctor as soon as possible.
If you tested positive, inform your friends and family immediately, take treatment as needed, and protect others from the contagion as best as possible.

DON'Ts

Don't smoke
Don't use opioid drugs
Don't become obese

Don't text and drive
Avoid alcohol addiction
Don't mix alcohol and medications
Don't drive under influence of alcohol or drugs
Don't drive while tired or sleepy
Don't speed or hurry when driving
Avoid road rage
Don't be greedy
Avoid arguments and those who irritate you,
don't say anything at all if you disagree
Don't use harsh words
You cannot control others- so control yourself.
Don't keep a gun in your house or your possession
unless highly skilled in its use
Don't participate in risky and adventurous activities
Don't walk outside without footwear
Avoid polluted areas and environments

Section 9- Immortality

Chapter 38

SEEKING IMMORTALITY

Upanishads are very ancient Hindu teachings and morals, written around 1000 BC. One of the stanzas is used in Hindu ceremonies and prayers even today. It says- Asatoma Sadgamaya, Thamasoma Jyothirgamaya, Mrithyoma Amirtham Gamaya. It translates as "Let falsehood be replaced by truth, let ignorance be replaced by knowledge and let death be replaced by immortality". The prayer carries a lot of meaning for all people in all times where the truth will eventually prevail, and education is the road map for one's future, and we seek immortality and make efforts to prolong life.

There has been a prolongation of life over the past century. People who used to die in their 40's are now living well into the '80s. The longest recorded longevity of humans is around 120 years. The longest recorded age is 122 set by Jeanne Calment of France. Many people are living well into their 90's and some are hitting 100 years of age. According to the US census bureau, there are 82,000 centenarians now in the US, and it is expected to be 140,000 in the next 10 years. The world's centenarian population is expected to grow eightfold by 2050. Those who are 65 years old today have a 50% chance that they will live to their 90s. The cancer death rate has come down by 26% compared to 1990. It estimated that a South Korean girl born in the year 2030 could expect to live to the age of 90.8. Statistics show that 10,000 people are turning to age 65 every day in the US and becoming new enrollees into Medicare. It is predicted that 30% of the US population will be above age 65 in the foreseeable future.

There is no doubt that life expectancy has almost doubled in the last 100 years. Still, the fact remains that death is inevitable, and there comes a day when the human body stops functioning. Older people have more disorders and chronic conditions requiring more medications and health care. 75% of people older than 65 have at least one chronic condition, and 20% of them have at least five chronic conditions. Now we know that certain items can prolong life. Nicotinamide containing compounds and telomerase enzyme inside the cell are two entities that prolong the life of chromosomes. This has been accomplished because of better health care, preventive medical measures, control of communicable diseases, availability of antibiotics and other wonder drugs, improved and advanced medical science, improved environmental conditions, and living conditions.

The quest for immortality is described from time immemorial. Ancient epic stories describe immortality is achieved by good individuals who lived a pious and saintly life with devotion to God and kindness to all living creatures. They become demigods also called Devas, as their souls go up to heaven upon death. Those who lived a sinful life, who were cruel to others and who did harm to others, had bad behavior and bad intentions were punished at death by sending their souls to hell. Either way, there was life after death and there was immortality to the soul, one went to a place of happiness, comfort, and luxury while the other went to a place of hardship, suffering, and manual labor.

Another quick route to attain immortality is also described in the epic storybooks. It is by drinking a special potion or nectar called Amritham. Mrtyu is the Sanskrit word for death. Amrit means the absence of death or immortality. The story goes on to describe that this particular nectar was highly sought after by the gods and devils because the person who drank it will attain immortality. The potion was hidden in the bottom of the earth beyond the seven seas. The fight between good and evil continues even today. These edicts are depicted as carvings on the walls of Angor Wat, an ancient temple in Cambodia. These carvings are estimated to be at least 2000 years old and are well preserved as UNESCO Heritage.

Immortality is assured and well known for unicellular organisms like bacteria and ameba. They can split themselves into two at their will any time and continue to live forever by multiplying over and over. They have the same chemicals or chromosomes in their cells as the original ones. As the creatures became multicellular they have the process of reproduction by combining the male spores or sperms with the female spores or ovum to create a new offspring. Even though they maintain the general features of the parents, the offspring are not the exact reproduction of the parents.

If we can specifically determine what leads to the death of the cell or what leads to the disruption of the chromosome inside the cell, we may be able to prolong the life of the cell and thus the life of the species. However, we still do not have a real answer to this except for some theories.

Similarly, medical science has not been able to create a living cell out of chemicals so far. We know the structure of the cell, what chemicals are in it, we know how to clone a cell, we know how to fertilize a cell inside the body as in vivo fertilization or outside the body as in vitro fertilization, we have DNA patterns and typing available, we know how a cell dies, but still, we have not been successful in creating a new cell de- novo from chemicals. If we can do that then we will become Gods, since that cell can be made to multiply.

Also, we do not know what is out in space or other planets for sure. We have some theories that may be right or wrong. We had certain opinions in the past that were proven wrong afterward. For example, we thought the earth was flat at one time and that the sun was rotating around the earth another time. Similarly, we think space is empty now, but there is proof to show that there are certain fine particles out there. There are many more solar systems and probably there is life in one or more of those distant planets. Just this month they discovered that 12 moons are circling Jupiter.

In the practical world, immortality is remembering certain special people for a long time after they have passed. Those individuals have made a major impact in society or to humanity as a whole. We know that Jesus Christ was a living legend. Many of the Hindu Gods such as Rama and Krishna were living humans at one time. Great emperors, founding fathers of nations, those who made monuments, wrote books, made scientific recoveries, made an impression in art, music, sculpture are all remembered.

As well, we have to ask what happens to a person's cell when an organ is donated to another person and that person lives for an extended period. Did the first person's cells live in another person and if so when did that person actually die? So a person can die but his or her organs can live longer.

A good theory is to clone oneself to remain immortal. When the cells age and begin to fail, create a new one. Cloning is a proven medical science but still has many hurdles to overcome. Stories of mythology have suggested cloning in ancient times, where a certain person can remain immortal by growing new body or body parts. Adolf Hitler had tried to clone his own body as shown in the movie Boys from Brazil. Cloning became a big story with the birth of Dolly, a lamb in 1967. Still, it involves a very tricky process of harvesting an egg cell, removing all the chromosomes from inside, harvesting a donor cell, injecting the donor nucleus back into the egg cell, and after it has grown to the tiniest embryo, implanting it inside a mother's womb and hoping for it to grow. In spite of all the excitement, cloning is still in infancy and is fraught with many problems, such as defective offspring, with degenerative diseases, and early death.

In cellular biology, we know of stem cells that can become any type of cell or organ from the embryonic pluripotent stem cells. In the commercial world, efforts are being made to produce artificial meat that looks and tastes the same as meat, but it is cultured from cells in the laboratory. They are called alternative meats or cultured meats or cell-based meats. They are made from starter cells from tissue extract and replicated in a protein medium inside the bioreactors. The meat that comes out will behave as meat from slaughtered animals, with the same nutrition and flavor.

There are many things probably unseen or undiscovered by humans, and these items may be true and existing around us. Just because we have not recognized it so far, we cannot categorically deny them as fake. As science advances, we accept them as true. We cannot deny the existence of the soul or the prime soul because we have yet to discover the very minute molecular particles or the largest entities in the universe begin.

There are many types of rays or waves that we cannot see, but we know that they exist and we can feel the effect. Radio waves, X-rays, Ultraviolet rays, television, and microwave are common today. We cannot see them, but we use them in everyday life. We can feel the wind, but cannot see it. God and the Universe are like that. The soul and prime soul are like that. We can feel the effect, but we cannot see them. We are part of it, with no beginning or end; we are a particle of it. Only the enlightened one can feel it, only those who use their extrasensory perception can feel the effect. It is like white light. You have to look through the prism to know that there are seven colors hidden inside the white light. You will wonder about the rainbow by not knowing the science behind it.

There is an everyday cycle on the surface of the earth which we take for granted, without seeing it. We see the rain, but we do not see the water vapor. We see the water in the ponds, lakes, rivers, and oceans, but do not see the vapor lifting up to the sky. We see the clouds and again see the rain coming down. Birth and death and the soul are like that. We see the death, but we do not see the soul-lifting up, and then we see the birth. Similar to the rainwater, birth and death are part of a cycle, in which the vapor and soul are not visible.

Much of it depends on how one thinks and sees. For some people, the universe is inert and random. For others, it is active and alive. Some want a scientific explanation and want proof of everything. Others are willing to accept the supernatural and the superior force above all. Features about the soul, God, or the prime soul are like that. It is a matter of how you see it, how you think about it, and how you accept it.

Ancient scriptures dictate that the body is made of five elements, namely earth, water, fire, air, and space or sky. We know of five senses namely touch, smell, hearing, vision, and taste. There may be other sensations and dimensions, which we do not know of. We see things in two or three dimensions, but there may be more dimensions, which we do not know of. Sometimes we call it a premonition or omen. There may be a sixth sense or extrasensory perception. We get a feeling of something that's going to happen before it happens.

Jose Luis Cordeiro and David Wood authored a book titled "The Death of Death". They describe a very possible scenario by which people can live 30 to 40 years longer than today with the further advent of stem cell therapy. Replacing old cells with new cells through stem cell therapy we may treat many of the aging problems and degenerative disorders and cancers. People will still die from accidents, suicides, and homicides. If we realize that humans are now living 30 to 40 years longer than they were living 100 years ago, it certainly stands to reason that they can live for another 30 to 40 years longer in the future also. There is a belief that many more incurable diseases today will become curable including cancers, dementia, Alzheimer's disease, heart attacks, and strokes. The aging process can be arrested or delayed. It may be possible to repair the telomeres in the chromosomes so that the chromosomes do not get disrupted so we can live for longer periods. It is the longevity of the chromosomes that keep the cells alive. The longevity of chromosomes is dependent on the longevity of telomeres and the enzyme called telomerase. It is already known that several techniques can increase the telomerase enzyme now.

We now know that certain individuals can recover miraculously after apparent clinical death. Certainly, the time posts and goalposts of defining death have changed. Comatose patients have regained normal function even after many months or even years. Heartbeats that stopped have regained the beats upon continuing CPR for an extended period. Until the soul finally departs, it still stays and wants to live. Life is possible after death until the soul agrees to leave.

By postponing the day of death we are attaining immortality by that many more days.

Chapter 39

IS THERE LIFE AFTER DEATH

Many people believe there is life after death either in the nether world or as reincarnation. There is a strong opinion that the soul or Atman is indestructible, permanent, and immortal. It enters into the young body at the time of birth after it discards an old and worn out body at the time of death, just as we change our clothes from an old and dirty one to a new and clean one. So goes the teaching of Bhagawat Gita the main Hindu scripture.

In his book "After Life" Hank Hanegraaf makes an analogy with a caterpillar and butterfly with life and afterlife. See the caterpillar crawling and then hibernating and then the beautiful butterfly emerges out of it as a total surprise, which flies around and brings joy to itself and others. The life of humans is like that. It looks as if we are suffering from the mundane burdens of life, but after death, there is an entrance to a new and breathtaking world. Even though the caterpillar is no more, it lives further in a more wonderful way. After death is the resurrection with majestic metamorphism of the soul into a better world of joy.

In his book "Life after Death" Deepak Chopra makes the analogy to water vapor. You see the drop of water, then it becomes invisible, but then it comes back to earth as rainfall. The water sometimes flows into the ocean, merging with the large body of water. Similarly, the soul is invisible, leaves the body, and then comes back to be born again in another body. Sometimes the soul merges with the supreme God. We see the water, but we do not see the water vapor. Similarly, we see life in this body, but we do not see the soul, but we know the water is going through different phases.

Garuda Purana is a series of scriptures in Hinduism that details out the sacrament duties and rituals one should observe following the death of a family member. The soul hangs around for several days waiting for the mourning, rituals, and sacrifices to the soul. Only after it has satisfied itself with the sincerity, love and formality and respect exhibited by the immediate family members, and conduct of ceremonies and rituals ordained and performed by the rest of the family members, and only then will it reach Moksha or its place in the heavenly body.

The resurrection of Christ and the fellow crucified victims are celebrated in Christianity at the time of Easter. Christ died accepting all the sins committed by fellow humans. HE came back alive after three days to bestow love and forgiveness on those who committed the crimes because they did not know their ignorance and sins. The belief is that drinking from the golden chalice from which Christ drank the wine at the last supper will give immortality. The search for that chalice continues. The Bible says, " I am the resurrection and the life. Whoever believes in me, though he dies, yet shall he live" John 11:25

Ancient Egyptians believed that life on planet earth is only a prelude to the real journey to the nether world. The full and real-life was thought to begin after death, so they built the pyramids with all the needed items for the journey in their tombstones, buried next to the mummified body of the Pharaoh or emperor. They placed pots and pans, utensils, fine clothes and jewelry, cows and goats, slaves and women, furniture and chariots, and other such things inside the tombstones.

The big question is for us to agree or disagree on whether there is a soul or not. Is it possible that the soul is just imagination or is it real? During our life, we agree that there is a mind, which is a function of the brain. The human brain is more advanced than the brain of other creatures. It can analyze, remember, and calculate. It has emotions and thinking capacity.

When the mind reacts, often we feel a choking sensation and we end up considering that the soul is in the chest next to the heart. We also assume that the seat of a person's soul is in the chest cavity at or near the heart. Many people say that they have seen the soul depart from the body in the form of flame coming out the chest or from the mouth at the time of death.

When we sneeze, we say "God bless you" or "bless you" or similar words in other languages and cultures. It originated a long time ago, with the thought that the soul would come out during the sneeze, and the devil could get in. The blessing was a way of warding off the evil and to protect the soul. During the sneezing one would tighten the chest muscles, hold the breath, and forcefully cough out through the nose, closing the eyes and pushing the tongue at the same time.

Hindus believe that the soul never dies and it joins a larger body of souls. The individual soul is called Atman and the larger body of the soul or the Primal soul is called Brahman. Atman is just a fraction of the Brahman. Brahman is the Supreme Soul, the creator of the universe, or God as we generally call Him. A certain Hindu prayer goes on to recite a stanza, which translates as " The Universe is infinite, God is infinite, but the infinite of the universe lies within the infinite of God, who created the infinite of the universe".

A question was asked if all the wealth of the entire world is to become mine, could I have immortality? The answer was no. Immortality is not delivered by wealth, but if you reach out to the soul inside of you and realize the God inside of you, reflect on Him and meditate on Him, you will identify with the Supreme Soul and will understand immortality.

The creation of the universe and the components of the universe is a mind-boggling phenomenon- how was it created and who created it. Even with the most advanced telescopes and technology we can see or fathom only a very tiny part of this universe that holds millions of the stars, suns, and planets.

The sun is the source of energy for the planet, the Sun God to whom people prayed from ancient times is depicted in the ancient holy prayer that goes like this: "The Sun is the sole source of energy, and let me derive inspiration from the Sun". The sun is 92,000,000 miles away from earth. To believe in God all you need is to look at the magnitude of the Sun and the universe and the God who created it. We, humans, are nothing but a speck of a particle in it.

The creation of the universe took many billions of years and is constantly changing and evolving. Scientific evidence shows there was a huge explosion, called the Big Bang, following which there was a massive cloud of dust and gas consisting of hydrogen, helium, and other elements, which became the Nebula. The condensation of the particles and gravity created the new stars and planets. As the stars eventually died after many more millions of years when the nuclear fusion in the core exhausted, the star collapsed pulling the gas inwards, causing a sharp bigger explosion, thus expanding and widening the universe and creating new stars and planets. Life on this planet is still evolving. Life on other planets is strongly considered as a possibility because the DNA is nothing but a few chemicals held together. These chemicals can change their configuration and create a different set of animals, with smarter brains than the human brain.

For God, there is no beginning and there is no end, He is all-encompassing, all-pervasive, all-inclusive, and supremely powerful. Yet we the humans think that we are smart. The unknowns are much more than the known.

The question was asked as to whether someone has seen the soul, or God, or the primal soul called Brahman. The answer was given in the following way. A pinch of salt was handed out and the person was asked to mix it with water in the ocean. The next day he was asked to return the pinch of salt. It was not to be seen. The seawater had a taste of salt before and after this pinch of salt was put in. You know the salt is in there; you can taste it but cannot see it. Yet by modern methods, you can recover some salt from the ocean, but the ocean water still tastes salty despite such recovery. The individual soul is just a speck of the Universal soul that we know exists, but cannot be seen.

The author wants to say that the Atman or individual soul is part of the Primal Soul or Brahman. You can say for sure that it is there and one can feel it if you look for it. Brahman is so vast and infinite and part of the Universe or part of God. Removing one soul or one pinch of salt is not going to diminish the God or infinity of the universe and it knows it will rejoin the universe when its role is over. The soul, which is the Lord within each person cannot die and does not age. It is part of the Supreme soul, which is everywhere, within all beings, all persons, vast and immortal and omnipotent and omnipresent.

Some people believe that the soul weighs 21 grams of weight. This is based on some observation that the weight of the body before death and immediately after death was lower by this amount. That is accounted for by the departure of the soul. It may be also due to the loss of water and body fluids too. Some people whom I have talked to including highly educated doctors and scientists believe in the soul, and its departure upon death and they also believe in reincarnation. They see a sudden flare-up of the face, rotation of the neck, and a brightness of the eyes or a spurt of energy just before death. They vouch to seeing or feeling the departure of the soul.

Hinduism links Karma to reincarnation. The good deeds done in this birth will bring in better fortune in the next life. A lady pediatrician tells me that it is the good deeds she did in the last birth that has brought good fortune and the good life in this current life. Bad deeds will result in punishment, poverty, or rebirth. Those who believe in reincarnation also think that rebirth is due to Karma or the deeds or behavior in this life. The soul can reincarnate also because it left behind an incomplete mission, it has a desire to spend more time, it has an attachment to worldly materials, or it is still bonding family members.

In the Hindu epic story of Mahābhārata, there are numerous examples quoted to explain birth and death. Many believe their lives are predetermined and preordained and destiny cannot be changed, even though ordinary people may question the rationale and unjust consequences. On certain occasions, two questions are asked- what is inevitable in life and what is the biggest wonder in life? The first question of what is inevitable is answered as death. The second question of the biggest wonder in life, it was answered that everyone thinks that death is not going to happen to them, but only to others.

However the ideal and ultimate goal is not to be reborn, but to be in Nirvana or Moksha or salvation. To achieve that, one has to be leading a very ascetic life, with total detachment from all worldly desires, as a saint. Alternately one should have served seven cycles of rebirths and suffered enough on this earth, and should pray to be liberated from further rebirths and sincerely seek salvation. It is also possible to get to Moksha or salvation by following one of the three Yoga lives (conduct of life) namely Bhakti Yoga, where one is deeply in prayer and devotion to the Lord, or Karma Yoga, where one is deeply involved in the best work possible, or Jnana Yoga, where one is having the divine knowledge and spirituality of highest order.

Discussion about the existence of heaven and hell is a time-honored argument that goes to prehistoric times. In Homer's Odyssey, the Greek hero Odysseus visits the underworld of dead people and sees the torture and torments of those who had offended the gods. They were doomed to harsh work as punishment and water and food were denied.

Christianity clearly defined the existence of the hell that was cruel and oppressive and the heaven for angels with softness and comforts. Hell is for Satan and Heaven is for angels and God. It is a clear-cut distinction.

This idea lost some acceptance with the advancement of scientific knowledge and Darwin's theories of evolution. However still even today, more than 50% of the population believes in heaven and hell according to a survey by Pew Research Center in 2014. Yet others have the opinion that heaven and hell are right here on the earth, making it a metaphor that those who committed crimes or bad deeds will pay for it one way or another.

Most scriptures, ancient epics as well as most people in today's world believe in heaven, which is an eternal world of peace and happiness and glory. The good souls go to this paradise. When asked, most people believe that heaven is somewhere up above us, pointing towards the sky, towards the solar system or universe. No one has seen it but the movies depict a glorious city located between clouds or higher up, where the inhabitants have wings and look like angels, who can fly and visit the planet earth at their will. It is the home of the Gods and Demi-Gods, angels, and spirituals. Certain religions such as Hinduism and Christianity depict God as having a human form. Islam and Jewish religions do not have a form or image for God. The Lord and angels are usually represented in white flowing robes while the demons, Satan, and evil are represented in black outfits with scary features.

As to what happens when one reaches heaven is described differently. Hindus have a view that everything is beautiful and pleasant over there. Everyone is gorgeous in their looks, with no blemishes, pimples, or scars. All have fabulous clothing, the weather is perfect, there is soft music all the time, women are dancing to entertain the audience, there is no hunger and there is no death or illness. Christians believe all their dreams come true in heaven. There is no misery, everyone is wearing pure white clothes, and they can fly like angels.

Therefore the question is where is heaven and how does one reach it? The ancient holy men and scriptures had an abstract sense of it. They said something like this: Maybe you are looking for heaven to feel the blissful experience. If you think it is in the skies, where Brahma resides, then birds that fly will be there before you. If you think it is in the sea where Vishnu resides beyond the seven seas, then fish that swims will be there before you. If you think it is in the mountains beyond the forests where Shiva resides, then animals that run fast will be there before you. If you are looking for bliss, then all you need to do is to reach inside of you. You will find your soul and spirit. It is in your kindness, conscious, and actions. You will find heaven and it is for you to experience it. It is up to you to feel the bliss.

By the same standards, hell is described as the place where evil-minded souls go after the death of human life. All scriptures describe hell as a place of eternal torture, pain, suffering, and horrific events. It is dark, foul-smelling with the noise of pain and suffering being heard. You are forced to work hard as if in jail. The sinners are expected to go to hell. Hell is dark, smelly, filled with snakes and scorpions, and is managed by equally dark sinister looking managers, who want to whip you, waterboard you, harass you and roast you up on fire or fry you in boiling oil. When asked most people say hell is below where we stand, meaning the center of the earth, which is hot and boiling.

Either hell or heaven, it is agreed by all that the soul separates and goes somewhere after death. This is described as life after death. Multiple polls show that 90% of people believe in heaven, but only 75% of people believe in hell. Most everyone believes in a soul, but they may give different interpretations as to how they define the soul.

What is the real effect of cosmic influence on our body and mind? What is the power of the sun on the genetics and behavior of humans? Are there particles from the solar system that are still undiscovered, smaller than the neutrons and protons, that are present in every living creature and affecting their lives? Do these particles form the soul and go back to the larger pool of particles? Do the planets influence what is to come?

The creation of each of us is also a phenomenon by itself, still poorly understood. If the matter can neither be created nor destroyed and if energy can neither be created nor destroyed, what happens to the human body, which is full of chemicals and full of energy? Does the mind possess energy? Can brain energy be transformed into other forms of energy? Is it true that psychics has the ability to see the ghosts and feel the foregone ones and hear their words? Is it all fake and illusion or there is an element of truth it?

When there is no evidence that any atom or molecule can reproduce itself or double on its own, how is it that a combination of some chemicals held in the DNA can double itself and carry within a set of codes to create new life. The human body is just a set of chemicals- 60% being water. Of the remaining 40%, it is 62% carbon, 11% nitrogen, 10% oxygen, 6% hydrogen, 5% calcium, 3% phosphorus, 1%pottasium, and 2% 28 different trace metals. It has not been possible so far to create life in a laboratory. Robots try to simulate humans but not in the real meaning of life. How do these chemicals add life to their combination? The seven aspects of life as we know are growth, reproduction, irritability, movement, excretion, nutrition, and death. (GRIM END) Can the machines become living creatures one day? Can we ever create life from chemicals one day?

There are many unanswered questions about life and death. Some things we know, but there are many things we do not know. Some are mythology, some are beliefs, and some may be outright false fiction, but just because we do not know or understand something today, it does not mean the truth will ever remain undiscovered.

About the Author

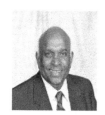 Dr. Venkit S. Iyer was born in Palghat District, Kerala State in India. The value of education was emphasized by the family from childhood, which helped him achieve higher education and admission to medical school there. After completing his medical degree, he did his post-graduation in surgery there. Immediately afterward he migrated to the United States for further training in surgery. After completing his internship and residency in New York, he started working at the same hospital as a full-time teaching faculty member in the department of surgery. After a year of work and teaching at Albert Einstein College of Medicine, Bronx, New York he decided to move to Florida to start a consulting practice in general and vascular surgery. After 30 years of active practice of surgery, he retired. Since then he has participated in various medical missions and charitable work. He also authored a textbook in surgery titled as "Decision Making in Clinical Surgery", published by J.P Brothers Medical publishers (jaypeebrothers.com)

Dr. Venkit S. Iyer is a board-certified surgeon, Fellow of the American College of Surgeons (FACS), Fellow of the Royal College of Physicians and Surgeons of Canada (FRCS-C), Fellow of the International College of Surgeons (FICS), and holds a Master's degree (MS) in surgery. He has held many leadership positions, teaching positions, and participated in various non-profit organizations. He has published several articles in professional journals and regular magazines and has given many talks and lectures in various forums.